Praise for Howard Brockman's
Essential Self-Care for Caregivers and Helpers

"Howard Brockman has created 'the manual' for any professional or nonprofessional caregiver who serves with the intention of making a difference without losing him- or herself in the process. This is a well-written book that will help anyone become more conscious of their empathic practice, teach them how to skillfully balance it and at the same time, not be overwhelmed by their vocation. A must read!"
DR. JOE DISPENZA, bestselling author of
Evolve Your Brain: The Science of Changing Your Mind
as well as *Breaking the Habit of Being Yourself:
How to Lose Your Mind and Create a New One*

"Howard Brockman provides an insightful, broad-ranging, sophisticated look at the way subtle energy affects the caregiving process and the well-being of the caregiver. This book offers spiritually and energetically cogent ways to promote corrective self-care in the midst of high-intensity giving, both the professional and personal kind. This is a strong mix of the theoretical and the practical."
BELLERUTH NAPARSTEK, LISW, Author of
Invisible Heroes: Survivors of Trauma and How They Heal,
and creator of the *Health Journeys* guided imagery series

"Brockman's *Essential Self-Care for Caregivers and Helpers* brings a bold new perspective to the age-old challenge to caregivers— how to stay well while attending to the suffering of others. He carves out a wide arc as he describes the myriad influences that can cause caregivers and helpers to slide into burnout and absorb toxic energies from those they help. Considerations of one's basic temperament along with innovative self-care strategies make this a must read book for professionals and home-based helpers alike."

DR. FRED GALLO, author of *Energy Psychology* and *Energy Tapping for Trauma*

"A wonderful book for anyone who cares for others. I found the advice to be insightful, thoughtful and compassionate. Keeping oneself in good mental health is critical for our well-being and those we care for. I think this will become a critical resource for caregivers. I highly recommend this as a book you keep close to your heart."

PROFESSOR ZORBA PASTER, University of Wisconsin School of Medicine and Public Health Host of public radio's *Zorba Paster On Your Health*

"For 40 years I have insisted to my patients that their primary responsibility is to take care of themselves FIRST so that they can help others. Health care personnel are just as much in need of SELF-Care, as their primary responsibility. Here is the foundation for all to heed!"

C. NORMAN SHEALY, M.D., PhD
President, Holos Institutes of Health
Professor Emeritus of Energy Medicine

"*Essential Self-Care for Caregivers and Helpers* will be just as helpful and relevant to the millions of baby boomers taking care of aging parents as to those in the helping professions. Howard Brockman emphasizes what too many people know yet tend to overlook—while helping others, one must still practice excellent self-care in order to stay well. He helps the reader understand vicarious trauma and how to distinguish its signs and symptoms from healthy stress. Helping doesn't have to be depleting or traumatizing as long as we understand how to create and maintain healthy boundaries. Brockman describes just how this is done. Congratulations for a job well done!"
SHARON CASS-TOOLE, PHD, Integrative Psychotherapist, Toronto, Canada

"Howard Brockman gives a great new spin to empowering the lives of caregivers. Working with energy psychology and core principles of consciousness, this book gives specific, useful examples of how to handle challenging situations and maintain your own healthy "home frequency." Brockman is a good writer, too! Easy to read and understand, with interesting case studies— this is a resource you'll want to keep near at hand."
PENNEY PEIRCE, author of *Frequency* and *The Intuitive Way*

"Howard Brockman has mined a wealth of cutting edge ideas and methods to pull together a useful and empowering guide for caregivers."
DAVID FEINSTEIN, PHD
Co-Author, *The Promise of Energy Psychology*

"Many thanks to Howard Brockman for his much needed, compassionate and thorough guidance in *Essential Self-Care for Caregivers and Helpers*. May we slow down long enough to absorb his deep wisdom and practice his excellent healing exercises. This book is for everyone who loves and works with others! Thank you Howard for the positive healing influence of your words and suggestions."

CAROL LOOK, LCSW, EFT MASTER,
Author of *Attracting Abundance with EFT*

Essential Self-Care for Caregivers and Helpers

Preserve Your Health,
Maintain Your Well-Being and
Create Effective Boundaries

Howard Brockman, LCSW

COLUMBIA

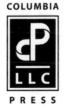

LLC

PRESS

Columbia Press LLC
1620 Commercial St. SE
Salem, Oregon 97302

Dynamic Energetic Healing® and are registered trademarks
of Howard Brockman and The
Heart Center Incorporated (an Oregon Corporation).

Editor: Linda Jenkins
Cover image: Willow Arlenea
Illustrations: Andrea Foust
Cover and book design: Jerry Soga
Composition: William H. Brunson Typography Services
Proofreader: Abigail Whitney

ISBN-13 978-0-9766469-4-5

Library of Congress Control Number 2012903611

To find out more about Howard Brockman's work and order books
directly from the publisher, go to: www.DynamicEnergeticHealing.com

Book Disclaimer

Howard Brockman

Essential Self-care for Caregivers and Helpers

The information contained in this book, including ideas, suggestions, remedies, approaches, techniques, methods, and other materials, is provided only as general information and is solely intended for your own self-improvement and is not meant to be a substitute for medical or psychological treatment and does not replace the services of health care professionals. If you experience any emotional distress or physical discomfort using any of suggestions, remedies, approaches, techniques, or methods contained in this book, you are advised to stop and to seek professional care, if appropriate.

Publishing of the information contained in this book is not intended to create a client-therapist or any other type of professional relationship between the reader and the author. The author does not make any warranty, guarantee, or prediction regarding the outcome of an individual using this book for any particular issue.

You agree to assume and accept full responsibility for any and all risks associated with using any of the suggestions, remedies, approaches, techniques and methods described in this book and agree to accept full and complete responsibility for applying what you may learn from reading this book. By continuing to read this book you agree to fully release, indemnify, and hold harmless, the author, and others associated with the publication of this book from any claim or liability and for any damage or injury of whatsoever kind or nature which you may incur arising at any time out of or in relation to your use of the information presented in this book. If any court of law rules that any part of the Disclaimer is invalid, the Disclaimer stands as if those parts were struck out.

DEDICATION

To my wife Anita and my sons, Noah and Elias,
whose experience of deep and enduring relationship
continues to nurture and support me.

CONTENTS

PREFACE

I have been in the helping professions since I began teaching at Oregon State University in Corvallis, Oregon, in the late 1970s. I had recently completed my master's degree in social ethics and religious studies at the University of Southern California in Los Angeles. I was unable to get a job in the greater L.A. area, so my wife, my new son and I decided to move to Oregon to escape the sprawling and smog-laden L.A. basin. I was twenty-six years old and had romantic aspirations of having a small farm in the country. My inner drive to pursue the subject areas of my master's program led me to a job in the Religious Studies department of Oregon State University, where I replaced a professor who was on sabbatical. For the next few years I taught small colloquia in the university honors program. I found this work very gratifying except for one thing—I had a strong desire to go deeper into the interpersonal context than the academic environment allowed.

Luckily for me, my application to the graduate School of Social Work master's program at Portland State University was accepted, and thus my professional direction shifted in a way that was more in alignment with my empathic temperament. By that time, I was teaching Kundalini Yoga and meditation classes and had opened a small private practice in Salem, Oregon.

This was a period of intense personal growth for me. I won't recount in detail all of the therapy and healing models that I pursued during this time, since that story is told in my first book, *Dynamic Energetic Healing*®. Suffice it to say that my appetite for expanding awareness was fairly insatiable. I spent two years studying gestalt therapy, three years learning Ericksonian hypnotherapy, ten years studying with Dr. Arnold Mindell to learn process-oriented psychology (also known as processwork), and in 1997 began my studies in energy psychology. In addition, during this period I began what turned into my thirty-plus years of studying and practicing core shamanism. During the first eight of those thirty-plus years, I was fortunate enough to be mentored in shamanic healing techniques by a woman who would later become a dear friend of mine.

In 1997, two colleagues and I began our several years of regular meetings to practice and integrate our energy psychology studies. We developed what emerged as Dynamic Energetic Healing®. I then went on to create my own synthesis, which I also refer to as DEH™. It integrates all the psychological and healing methods that I learned previously, in particular, core shamanic practices, energy psychology applications and processwork principles.

Various forms of talk therapy tend to monopolize Western approaches to psychotherapy and counseling, thanks to the biased view that rational insight into problem states is the best avenue to resolve clients' presenting problems. Thanks to my early interest in learning non-Western approaches to *healing* (yes, this is what non-Western people call the outcome of what we call therapeutic intervention) and my rigorous Western graduate school training, I was drawn to develop and synthesize a healing model that fits incredibly well into a Western-based psychotherapeutic context.

From the beginning, I have been using and teaching DEH as the organizing framework for my therapeutic healing model. I had not thought about writing my first book, *Dynamic Energetic Healing*®, until I started having remarkable therapeutic outcomes with the people I worked with using DEH. These successes inspired me to write case study summaries of sessions that I had with clients just because I had to get them down in print. Later, when I was teaching DEH to other therapists, it dawned on me that the training materials I was writing had the potential to expand into a book. I decided that I had a lot to say about why this model works so effectively. It took about four years to put this all together, and *Dynamic Energetic Healing*® was published in 2006. It has won four publishing awards and continues to sell regularly in the United States, Europe and Russia.

As I recount in Chapter 12, soon after I began studying the energy psychology model intensely I came down with a mysterious exhaustion that persisted for a number of years. I became gradually more fatigued during my workweek, and was so exhausted by Friday evening that I was frequently bedridden throughout the weekend. The deep ache in my kidney/adrenal area (in the mid- to low back) precluded any kind of sustained activity. With bed rest and minimal weekend activity, my energy was sufficiently restored to be able to get back to work on Monday, when the cycle began again. This pattern went on for a number of years, until I went to Brazil in 2003 to seek healing from a man named John of God. In our first meeting, he told me that I was absorbing the energies of my clients. Through various means during the two weeks I was there, I was healed of this condition completely. This experience was a contributing factor motivating me to write my first book.

Since that time, both in my teaching seminars and in my private practice, I have noticed that many of my clients and trainees who are therapists or helpers have similar issues with ongoing exhaustion. I became curious about related phenomena that are reputedly the causes of what is called compassion fatigue and caregiver burnout. I began to research the literature on these topics. I discovered that while there are commonly accepted themes related to the issue of compassion fatigue, an entirely different dimension within the helping and caregiving relationship was not being addressed.

Because of the various spiritual and energy-based practices that I have learned over the years and continue to practice, I have developed heightened sensitivity to what I call subtle energies that are always being exchanged in the interpersonal context. Learning and applying energy psychology strategies in my DEH model essentially forced me to confront my lack of awareness of these interpersonal energetic exchanges, which were the cause of my ongoing exhaustion. As my own awareness became more heightened and inclusive over time, it became increasingly evident to me that this growing awareness and knowledge needed to be communicated to others in the helping and caregiving fields.

Having said that, I wrote *Essential Self-Care for Caregivers and Helpers* for anyone who finds himself or herself in a helping or caregiving role. Foremost among this very large group of caregivers and helpers are nonprofessionals who find themselves in this role without any prior training. As an example, when a dying family member needs hospice care at home, usually a nurse helps establish the necessary home setup, which may include a hospital bed, a wheelchair and a medication management schedule. It then defaults to the family members to actually perform the care, including administering medications and looking after the bathing and toileting needs of the loved one. While the nurse will typically check in once a day or so, the majority of care is left to the family members, most of whom have had no preparation or training in the practical matters required for the care, let alone the emotional demands of day-to-day caretaking responsibilities.

If you are one of the many millions of baby boomers who are taking care of an aging parent, you will find this book as helpful and relevant as those who make their living supporting and helping others. In fact, as a nonprofessional caregiver who has been recruited by your family to help an ailing parent, you will find this book especially useful. You may be least prepared to consciously consider issues of secondary traumatization or compassion fatigue, and in some ways you are especially prone to the potential hazards of helping. The old, persistent dynamics and relational patterns of your family tend to generate internal conflict and resentments for you and the parent you are caring for. It's often very difficult to continually attend to someone from the place of heartfelt compassion if you feel you have been neglected, unsupported, criticized or abused by that person. These family dynamics create even greater challenges to establishing and maintaining proper energetic boundaries (see Chapter 7) when dealing with an abusive or critical parent. Maintaining your health and well-being under these circumstances becomes particularly challenging.

Many people today accept that there is a complex relationship between their mind and body. Thus, they acknowledge that psychosomatic symptoms, such as the common cold, a migraine headache or a stomach ache, can be caused by stress. We are also beings with an incredibly powerful consciousness that is always connected to others. This power, which many people are unaware of, far exceeds our rational thinking brain in terms of its ability to influence events and other people. Consequently, there is much that we can do to support others by integrating our thinking and intent with an attitude of compassion. We can have profound positive and healing influences when we become aware of this aspect of ourselves and learn to be more deliberate and conscious in its application.

I address these issues and others in *Essential Self-Care for Caregivers and Helpers*. It is my hope that by reading this book, you will more consciously continue to support others and, at the same time, become more successful in taking care of yourself.

ACKNOWLEDGMENTS

First and foremost, I want to acknowledge all the clients and students in my training program who, over many years, have shared their struggles and revealed the emotional difficulties they've been challenged with from taking care of and helping others. They have included fellow therapists, counselors, psychologists, social workers, hotline workers, nurses, doctors, ministers, teachers and school administrators. The list also includes the many nonprofessional helpers and caregivers who have found themselves assisting and taking care of their aging parents even though they never signed on for this demanding task. Every one of them has taught me so much and inspired me to think more deeply about the common themes, issues and consequences that emerge from assisting and helping others. I thank you all for challenging me to better understand and articulate the many ways that we can continue to be helpful while preserving our health and maintaining our own well-being. Certainly this remains a challenge for all of us.

This book would not have been possible without the remarkable talent and skill of Linda Jenkins, my editor. Linda was instrumental in helping me shape the manuscript into a tight, cohesive structure, helping me connect disparate ideas to come together with wonderful fluidity, and gently offering suggestions when necessary, all while supporting my vision unconditionally with professional expertise and commitment. Writing can be a very solitary experience, and to have an editor who shared my enthusiasm for this project was a collaboration of the highest order.

Big thanks also go to my wife, Anita, whose great passion for life always inspires me to do my very best to find out what is possible.

CHAPTER

1

Being a Caregiver

Our society recognizes many people as being professional helpers or caregivers. As you will see below, they include a wide diversity of professions, including the following:

- Massage therapists, doctors, nurses, physical therapists, naturopaths and chiropractors support people by directly addressing their physical pain and bodily imbalances.
- Social services workers, including social workers, child welfare workers, legal aid lawyers, and employees of government organizations, help people obtain food stamps and housing and help them navigate the bureaucracies of the social safety net.
- Psychologists, hospice workers, counselors and psychotherapists, pastors, rabbis and ministers support the emotional and spiritual needs of their clients.

People in these helping professions spend a great deal of their time interacting with their clients. The context for their work is in the relationship—that's where they're engaged. Unlike computer programmers, who spend most of their time in front of a video monitor, or architects, who are absorbed in creating intricate building designs, helpers and caregivers are directly involved with people for a significant amount of their time.

But millions of other people in our society could become or are nonprofessional helpers or caregivers:

- Many of the over seventy-eight million baby boomers in the United States[1] now find themselves attending to the needs of their aging parents. With better healthcare technology and pharmaceutical drugs, Americans are living longer than ever before. This challenging reality is growing, as there is one American turning sixty years old every ten seconds!
- Homeless shelters, food banks and other community organizations are staffed primarily by volunteers.
- Parents of children who have disabilities (physical, mental or cognitive), or of teenagers who have drug problems, also fall into this category.

While the specifics of what each category of professional and nonprofessional helper does are unique, and while helpers have different training and expertise (or, in the baby boomer example, lack of any specific training), they do share a fundamental commonality—inherent in their role is *intense human contact driven by extraordinary need.* Therefore, although this book focuses on those who help for a living, our discussion of the challenges faced by caregivers and suggestions for how to meet these challenges are equally relevant to nonprofessional helpers.

All helpers are "high-intensity relaters"

I have coined the term *high-intensity relater* to designate helpers or caregivers—both professional and nonprofessional—who work in focused and sustained interpersonal helping contexts. I am a professional high-intensity relater—my currency is relationship and I am paid to help. There are millions of professional high-intensity relaters just like me—our vocation is helping others in all kinds of ways.

There are also millions of nonprofessional high-intensity relaters in America today. To reiterate the point made above, in many ways the experiences of a professional helper (such as a domestic relations mediator who is exposed to the psychotoxic anger of two acrimonious spouses) are fundamentally the same as the experiences of the parents of the teenager who is struggling with drug addiction. Although these situations are completely different, the mediator and the parents are all high-intensity relaters. They all ask themselves, "How can I help?"

What distinguishes high-intensity relaters from others is the degree to which they are engaged in the interpersonal context. While it may seem more apparent to you that a social worker doing home healthcare visits certainly qualifies as a high-intensity relater, so too does the pastor who counsels bereaved family members after a death, listening compassionately to their story about that person's life in order to speak to the congregation about the deceased during the

> I have coined the term *high-intensity relater* to designate helpers or caregivers—both professional and nonprofessional—who work in focused and sustained interpersonal helping contexts.

memorial service to follow. The lawyer who negotiates custody and visitation agreements between separating spouses is very much a high-intensity relater, but her colleague in the same law firm who spends all her days in the law library researching contracts for established precedents is not—she is not regularly engaged in the interpersonal context with clients. Similarly, clinical psychologists who spend their time engaged with clients all the time are high-intensity relaters, but psychologists who spend most of their time in an academic research setting are not.

To give you another example, let's look at two baby boomers, Dave and Bill, who are both responsible for assisting their elderly parents. Dave may only visit them twice a week to make sure their bills are paid and their checkbook is balanced. If he notices that a showerhead is leaking, he calls the plumber and arranges for an appointment to repair it. Dave is not a high-intensity relater. Meanwhile, Bill visits his elderly parents every day, makes sure they take all their medications, gets them up for short walks outside the house, and makes sure that they're clean and showered every day. Since he is with them on a daily basis, he hears about their aches and pains and bears witness to their physical disabilities. He is emotionally more plugged in to his parents' day-to-day problems than Dave is. Bill is a high-intensity relater. The essential difference between Dave and Bill is that the latter has ongoing engagement in the interpersonal context. It doesn't matter that Bill hasn't been professionally trained for his role as caregiver, or that he never planned (or even wanted) to take on that role.

It is important to note that although Bill and millions of others are "recruited caregivers," their consuming role in an interpersonal context makes them just as much high-intensity relaters as those who choose to join a caregiving profession and those who actively choose to become nonprofessional caregivers.

Thus, regardless of your station in life, if you are in a situation of intense interpersonal contact, whether it be from choosing your vocation as a profession or quite suddenly discovering that you are needed as a helper or caregiver, you will find this book to be a helpful guide for your self-care.

How helping affects high-intensity relaters

Most people recognize that receiving help from another person is an affirming, deeply satisfying experience. But what of the person who does the helping? What kind of experience is it for them? And why do some individuals, such as counselors, therapists, teachers and legal aid lawyers, dedicate their lives to helping others?

There are a plethora of reasons why some people, including me, choose to go into the helping or caregiving professions, or to be a nonprofessional helper (a voluntary caregiver). I believe that, fundamentally, it could be that we rediscover our essential nature when we are in communion with another person. The satisfaction that we derive from a helping or caring interaction moves us into a space (albeit temporarily) of deep personal satisfaction that in many cases opens us up to greater compassion. It is during these brief moments that there is a deep communion of essence to essence, a mutual rapport that transcends class, rank or position.

Perhaps the helping context is our most direct route to being at peace and harmony with ourselves and with our outer environment, which includes other people, other life forms, the earth and our local community.

To enable us to survive in our increasingly complex, fast-paced society, our attention has become very externally driven and outer directed. As a result, we end up with multiple layers, one upon the other, of psychological and emotional defenses. With the wounding that happens just by being human (i.e., having to experience our own and other people's suffering), we acquire and develop multiple compensations in the way we think, feel, behave and interact with others. We mostly live day to day in a fear-based, overly vigilant state of consciousness. For most of us, this becomes our primary identity structure without our even being consciously aware of it.

But when high-intensity relaters focus their attention on helping another person, they move out of this overly vigilant state into an almost magical interactive trance in which one soul recognizes another. On one level the helper is "just doing their job," but at a much deeper level an energetic phenomenon is occurring. I call this phenomenon the *contagion of healing release into the sea of calm*. Many people simply call this experience love. As the helping facilitator opens herself to this communion of deep healing and compassion, she floats in this sea of calm. And the more she does this, the more benefits accumulate to her soul.

Some people describe the phenomenon of being in this sea of calm as "getting in touch with the Mind of God." Quantum physicists call it "connecting to the Unified Field." Meditation is one way to move into that place of unbounded awareness with a diminished sense of self-consciousness that emphasizes our sense of just being. Ancient spiritual masters taught that experiencing this state is the fruit of many years of disciplined spiritual practices. I believe that this state is also reached by caregivers when they experience this state of communion and deep rapport with the people who they help.

I have come to know this healing release through the guidance of my higher Self, and have corroborated it empirically when working with clients using my Dynamic Energetic Healing® protocol. (See Appendix 1 for more information on Dynamic Energetic Healing®.) I have learned that of all the benefits of being a high-intensity relater, this deeply spiritual experience is at the very core. This is the dimension of healing that reveals itself to the helper or caregiver as a blessing that can only come from being highly conscious. This is what keeps me coming back to help and what inspires me to write and to teach others how to facilitate within the interpersonal context. This is where profound pain is identified and released, so that suffering diminishes and new choices avail themselves—this profound experience allows dreams to be realized.

Based on my own experience and the experiences of many others, I know that the journey to reach the sea of calm is much like the mythic hero's journey—it is fraught with peril for the uninitiated. Like the Sirens' song that almost drove Odysseus and his crew to madness, caregivers encounter many seductions, obstructions and blind spots along the path to supporting those who need their help. Chapter 2 describes the rich and complex component of the human experience known as empathy. It is through empathy that one can experience the communion of deep healing and compassion, or can find oneself being dashed upon the rocks by the seductions of the Sirens' song.

Some people are involuntary high-intensity relaters

To be fair, we must acknowledge that many people who are in the caregiver role have not chosen it. Many of these "involuntary" high-intensity relaters do not experience that wonderful communion with others whom they are helping, or if they once did, they no longer do. They often find themselves resenting the needs of the people they are helping. Compassion fatigue and progressive burnout, which are discussed later in this chapter, are all about cumulative overwhelm.

For most of us, even though we may be dedicated to and feel fulfilled in our role as a caregiver, there comes a point when our threshold for attending to another begins to collapse. This happens to seasoned therapists, nurses and emergency medical technicians, as well as to adult children who are doing everything they can to support their aging parents. Being in a state of flow and compassionate rapport is a wonderful and sometimes transporting experience that evolves into a unique and personally fulfilling interpersonal dance. But the reality is that unless you are consciously *and regularly* working on a self-care regimen, you may gradually become less enthusiastic and more resentful toward the people you are trying to help. This is true for all professional and nonprofessional caregivers, whether they chose to be in their role voluntarily or were "drafted" by family circumstances or other factors.

> Unless you are consciously *and regularly* working on a self-care regimen, you may gradually become less enthusiastic and more resentful toward the people you are trying to help.

The expectation in a clinic, for example, is that the professional caregivers who work there are available to everyone who walks through the door, hour after hour, day after day. At the same time, due to concerns about professional liability, paperwork and documentation must be assiduously managed. Scheduling and organizing one's personal time for reflection and rest in that type of environment frequently become more difficult as the demanding needs of others persist. As a result, some professional caregivers who began their careers loving their jobs find themselves, years later, feeling frustrated, resentful and ready to quit.

Rafael

Let's look at the plight of Rafael. During college, he realized that he wanted to be in a profession that helped those in the community who had less advantages than many others. He was somewhat idealistic, but felt a strong conviction that working in a public health setting that served everyone, regardless of income, resonated with his deeper value system. He enjoyed interacting with people, and thus decided to get a master's degree in counseling.

During his practicum, Rafael was placed in a Catholic community services counseling clinic, where he learned a lot about family counseling and working with the homeless. He loved his work and received positive evaluations from his supervisor. In fact, his supervisor suggested that after he graduated he come to work at the clinic. Rafael was flattered and decided to accept the offer. Six weeks after he graduated he had his first job.

Fast-forward fifteen years—Rafael was now the clinic supervisor. His responsibilities included providing the direct service to clients that he initially enjoyed so much, plus overseeing and supervising five counselors and community volunteers, and writing grant proposals to solicit funding for the clinic. Rafael had grown into the job and embraced his many and varied responsibilities. He was a devoted father and husband as well as a committed clinic supervisor.

But something was not quite right. At night, Rafael was frequently unable to sleep. He was preoccupied with concerns about getting sufficient funding for the clinic, and the clients' needs kept increasing—more and more people were coming in for help after losing their jobs, marriages, or even their homes. Rafael was sensitive, and he was becoming increasingly aware of the desperation that many clients expressed about their lives. He frequently saw clients himself since the clinic could not afford to hire any additional counselors, and he was committed to not turning anyone away. All of his hired staff had full caseloads and many of them needed supervision and support from him in order to maintain their own sense of balance and harmony.

Soon, Rafael began to notice he was tired by lunch, so he started drinking more coffee. Although he didn't want anyone to know, he had already driven himself to the emergency room twice for what he thought were heart attacks, but that were found to be panic attacks. Rafael was feeling increasingly overwhelmed emotionally by the demands of his job, and eventually, he made an appointment with his doctor. After some tests, he was told he was suffering from adrenal exhaustion, and that drinking more coffee would actually exacerbate the condition. The doctor told Rafael that he needed to take a leave of absence in order to get a handle on his health. He was prescribed Zoloft for his panic attacks and another pharmaceutical drug to help him to sleep at night.

Rafael, who always enjoyed coming to work, was starting to resent the demands he had to deal with every day because he was unable to maintain his own physical and emotional health. He had chosen his profession for himself, and although he enjoyed the challenges, the clients, and his staff, he was starting to spiral downward into the vortex of feeling exhausted and depleted. He was unable to do his job and simultaneously take care of himself. The situation was starting to compromise his health, and he would potentially face dire consequences if he did not make a significant change. He felt stuck, and he was burning out.

Unfortunately, Rafael's case is all too common, particularly with the enormous federal and state deficits that are now eroding what was for many years ample funding for state and community mental health clinics.

But you don't need to be a professional caregiver or helper to find your ability to care for yourself compromised. Let's look now at a nonprofessional caregiver.

Janine

My client Janine is a caregiver to her mother, who is in her nineties and lives alone in her house in the Midwest. Janine shares the caregiving responsibility with her younger brother and older sister, who both live within driving distance of their mother. Janine's father died a few years ago, leaving her elderly and infirm mother alone in her house. Although her mother is mentally sharp, she cannot clean her house and has problems getting around to bathe and cook for herself.

Janine cares very much about her mother and wants the best for her. Janine has flown from her home on the west coast to the Midwest several times to discuss with her brother and sister how best to assist their mother. Not surprisingly, how much money and whose money to spend on her mother's care have been major issues of sibling contention. Even though Janine is now retired, she tries to send at least $400 toward her mother's care every month. She and her husband feel as though they have mortgage payments again, even though they recently finally paid off the mortgage on their home.

Janine frequently has acrimonious e-mail exchanges with her sister, who does not want to contribute any money to help their mother. She is stingy and controlling, particularly in relation to financial support issues. Janine's brother has medical problems that prevent him from being involved with his mother's care.

Amidst all these ongoing stressors and frustrations, Janine feels that, since she lives so far away, it is her duty to call her mother every evening in order to be supportive. These calls typically last from forty-five minutes to an hour. This is putting a strain on Janine's marriage because her husband complains that he now comes second and says that Janine is frequently depressed and upset after these nightly calls. Her husband feels shut out and ignored much of the time, and Janine feels distraught and increasingly depleted emotionally from her duties as a caretaker from afar.

Janine feels good about doing what she can to help her mother, but she's feeling overwhelmed by the nightly phone calls, the regular blaming and accusatory e-mails from her sister, and the frustration and complaints from her husband. Janine feels caught in the middle, just as countless other members of the baby boom generation who are in similar situations do.

The risks of being a high-intensity relater

As I have suggested, the rewards of caring for and helping others are many. They include (but are not limited to) positive shifts in one's value system, including greater tolerance and patience for other people; increased self-awareness; the experience of deep interpersonal connections with those being helped; a deepening of empathy along with increasing acceptance of differences without judgment or criticism; and greater tolerance for and acceptance of ambiguity.

However, as we've seen from Rafael's and Janine's stories, that is not the whole picture. Since all emotions are contagious, caregivers are at risk of becoming infected by the suffering of the person they're close to or attending to frequently. I don't know if this is a new concept to you but it's absolutely true! We "catch" other people's emotional energy in a way that's similar to how we catch their cold germs. (This is explained further below.)

> Since all emotions are contagious, caregivers are at risk of becoming infected by the suffering of the person they're close to or attending to frequently.

Even if it makes sense to you that being around someone who has a wasting disease—whether a patient in a hospital or a loved one at home—can be emotionally depleting and physically exhausting, you still need a great deal of self-care awareness to protect yourself against vicariously experiencing the other person's pain and suffering in your own nervous system. Upon reflection, you might think that this sounds logical for healthcare workers (or family members) who are attending to patients with a serious illness, but secondary traumatization and compassion fatigue affect people in many professions.

11

Let's look at lawyers, for example. Recent studies indicate that increasing numbers of attorneys who work with trauma victims have a surprisingly high rate of secondary traumatization symptoms. In addition to having higher rates of suicide and substance abuse than the general public, lawyers are also four times more likely to suffer from depression than the general public.[2] I think you'll agree that many lawyers qualify as high-intensity relaters.

But many other people also work in environments where people are in crisis or a great deal of despair. Some examples include the local banker who has to tell people that the bank is foreclosing on their home; the bus driver for a retirement community whose patrons are alone, frail and frequently ill; the 911 operator who receives calls from frightened citizens who are the victims of domestic violence; and the police officer who must interact with the families of people who have just been killed in an accident or a shooting. My point is that if you are in any line of work in which you interact with people who are vulnerable, suffering or in extreme emotional states, it's essential that you learn how to manage your own feelings of despair, fear, anger and hopelessness. Helpers and caregivers come into contact with these feelings every day.

Unfortunately, the very real challenges of caring for and helping others are often overlooked or minimized. However, the larger therapeutic community acknowledges that there are four primary risks that helpers and caregivers are vulnerable to. In addition, although it is not usually mentioned by the larger therapeutic community, I have added another type of risk, which I call *psychotoxic contamination.* This term refers to caregivers "catching" or becoming infected by the negative energy of the person they are caring for.

> Unfortunately, the very real challenges of caring for and helping others are often overlooked or minimized.

Keep in mind that these terms frequently overlap. Although healthcare professionals sometimes argue about which term is more appropriate to describe a specific circumstance, these terms and descriptions are often used interchangeably—they all describe what happens when individuals are around other people who are suffering and in pain.

In 1978, the term *burnout,* which was then associated with mental health workers, was first mentioned as a very real consequence of being a caregiver.[3] The symptoms of burnout are varied and complex. They include physical complaints, such as exhaustion, migraine headaches, chronic upper respiratory infections and irritable bowel syndrome, and various forms of mental and emotional anguish, such as depression, general feelings of overwhelm and chronic low-grade anxiety. In addition, burnout often results from a person working in an environment characterized by institutional constraints and administrative demands. If the person is unable to achieve their work-related goals in that environment over a long period of time, she gradually develops strong feelings of cynicism and frustration. A common consequence of this is a growing feeling of detachment from one's work and one's relationships at work and at home. Feeling burned out progressively erodes one's motivation to continue working in a job that was once gratifying and sustaining.

> I have added another type of risk, which I call *psychotoxic contamination.* This term refers to caregivers "catching" or becoming infected by the negative energy of the person they are caring for.

In 1985, the term *vicarious traumatization* appeared in an article in a therapy journal. The term was used to describe children who are profoundly negatively affected—even traumatized—by being around others (especially family members) who are experiencing physical, mental or emotional trauma or abuse. For the first time, research began to confirm the devastating effects experienced by people who simply witness other people's cruelty and pain.[4] For example, there is a significant likelihood that a child who witnesses her father regularly hitting and threatening her mother will be vicariously traumatized. Similarly, a customer in a convenience store who, although not directly threatened himself, witnesses a robber point a gun at the clerk's head is also highly likely to experience vicarious traumatization. Although one situation is repeated over time and the other is an isolated incident, both witnesses are at a high risk of vicarious traumatization.

As research into the effects of trauma began to proliferate, the term *secondary traumatization* emerged. This is an intersubjective (i.e., shared nonverbally between two or more people) or energetic phenomenon that is well documented in families and among caregivers and helpers. In a family context, an example would be when the major breadwinner loses his or her job because, say, the corporate owners outsource the position to China. With no immediate job prospect in sight, the breadwinner's self-identity and self-esteem are shockingly and irretrievably squashed. Aside from the financial consequences, everyone in the family experiences secondary traumatization as they become infected by the pervasive feelings of loss, anger and hopelessness that are omnipresent in the family field.

The fourth common phrase that's used interchangeably with the other three risks or "costs of caring" is *compassion fatigue.* This term was used as far back as the early 1950s among nurses who began to exhibit various symptoms of stress and diminished productivity accompanied by a pervasive negative attitude toward their work. However, it wasn't until 1995 that psychologist Charles Figley published a book on the ramifications of compassion fatigue.[5] Figley used this term to describe a condition characterized by a gradual diminishment of compassion over time. Those who suffer from compassion fatigue experience numerous symptoms, including hopelessness, anhedonia (decreased ability to experience pleasure), ongoing stress and anxiety, and a pervasive negative attitude that can lead to feelings of professional insufficiency or inadequacy. Essentially, compassion fatigue is synonymous with secondary traumatization.

At a fundamental level, your job as a caregiver is to be supportive and nonjudgmental toward the person you are helping. You do this in order to assist and provide counsel and healing for people who are bereft of resources (physical, mental, spiritual and/or financial) and need someone to help them deal with their limitations. After a session with a client or an afternoon with the family member you are caring for, you may feel depleted and drained. Many people in this situation assume that this drained feeling is the result of them expending their energy in order to help the other person.

But there is another explanation for this feeling—one that arises from viewing the situation from an energetic perspective. Rather than seeing the situation as one in which your energy level is affected but the other person's is not, this perspective recognizes that energy is in fact *being exchanged* between you and the other person. At the same time that you are depleting your own energy in order to help them, you are "picking up" some of their energy. The

> This perspective recognizes that energy is in fact *being exchanged* between you and the other person.

energy that you absorb from them has the capacity to be supportive or damaging to you. I use the term *psychotoxic contamination* to describe the situation in which one person (for example, the caregiver) picks up damaging or toxic energy from another (the person they are caring for).

Although you may be unfamiliar with the concept of energy exchange, this phenomenon is an empirically based reality reinforced by decades of well-grounded experimental research (see Chapter 4). On an experiential level, you may also be aware that some people are toxic to you because they emanate psychotoxic thoughts and energy. In most cases, much of that psychotoxicity is generated by them unconsciously, from the wounded part in them created and maintained from unhealed trauma.

The author's personal experience

In my first book, *Dynamic Energetic Healing®: Integrating Core Shamanic Practices with Energy Psychology Applications and Process-work Principles*, I explained how I found myself progressively physically depleted for a number of years when I was first learning energy psychology applications.[6] At first, I attributed this to the intense ongoing trainings I was participating in. Yet, none of my friends and colleagues who were participating in the same trainings complained about the fatigue and exhaustion that was plaguing me. As I discuss in more detail in that book (and in Chapter 12 here), I eventually discovered when visiting the healer John of God in Brazil that I had been absorbing the energies of my clients. This had never happened to me prior to my immersion into energy psychology, even though by that time I had already been a therapist in private practice for sixteen years. During those sixteen years, I had done just fine managing the potential hazards of emotional contagion, but my introduction into the energy psychology model (in which I was now working) had somehow left me too open and vulnerable to the toxic energies of my clients. Forced to inquire deeply into the nature of what had become a mysterious chronic fatigue, I discovered that there are other dimensions operating in the helping and caregiving relationship that I had previously been unaware of. In fact, there is a mosaic of personality traits or types—a composite, if you will that predisposes helpers and caregivers to fall under the spell of another.

The purpose of this book is to give you, the high-intensity relater, the tools you need to recognize, acknowledge and manage the feelings of despair, fear, anger, resentment, hopelessness and overwhelm that are frequently an inherent part of your role as a caregiver. In subsequent chapters, I explain the debilitating effects of unconscious empathy and how to establish solid energetic boundaries that will protect you from the emotional contagion that can be like catching the flu.

In many ways, this book expands on many of the innovatively effective approaches that are usually recommended to caregivers by practitioners of my Dynamic Energetic Healing® model (see Appendix 1). Here, these strategies are applied specifically to the problems experienced by high-intensity relaters. The result is an enormously expanded therapeutic paradigm that considers what is necessary in order for high-intensity relaters to sustain their health and well-being while supporting others in need. *Essential Self-Care for Caregivers and Helpers: Preserve Your Health, Maintain Your Well-Being and Create Effective Boundaries* expands on the trauma-based interventions discussed in my first book by considering the challenges to caregivers in all walks of life, and by providing a range of concrete strategies and approaches you can use to maintain your physical, emotional and spiritual health while you perform your caregiving role.

Questions and Exercises

1. To what degree are you a high-intensity relater? Is it your basic nature to be emotionally sensitive all the time? Or do you "turn on" this quality only when you are relating with others as part of your job? If you're only very sensitive at your job, do you feel this way only occasionally and intermittently? Or is it sustained and inherent in your work whenever you're interacting with others in a helping capacity? Answering these questions honestly should help you determine where you are on the "relating to others" continuum.

2. Caring for and helping others can compromise your health and well-being. Do you identify with any of the symptoms of burnout or compassion fatigue described in this chapter? If

so, I suggest that you make a list right now of any of your stress symptoms that might fit into these categories. Consider physical complaints that may now be chronic, and think about your mood, both during the time you're at work and the time when you're away from work.

3. Do you struggle with addiction to alcohol or other substances, including food? Even if you love your job, do you feel inordinate stress associated with it? Consider that your stress symptoms, which could include these substance addictions, carry important information that is connected to parts of your self that you may have lost touch with. Take an honest inventory of your relationship to alcohol, food and other substances. Is your relationship with any of these substances out of your control to some degree? Or do you feel uncomfortable about your relationship with that substance? If you answered yes to any of these questions, consider which part of you (that may not be getting enough attention) is crying out to you for help. Apply to yourself the skills that you use to help others—help that part of you that might be acting out through these stress symptoms or addictive propensities. Enter into a dialogue with it and find out what it needs. Perhaps a change in your daily life is now required.

4. Have you created a self-care program for yourself? Think about the ways in which you care for yourself as pieces of a puzzle. Do all your pieces fit together? What pieces may be missing? For instance, you may be committed to a regular exercise program to maintain your physical fitness. But do you have a healthcare professional with whom you meet regularly, or do you only see your doctor when you have a problem or an emergency? If you are strategic about developing and maintaining your self-care program, you will find that the pieces of the puzzle will evolve to complement each other into an integrated

whole. Optimal self-care doesn't just help you stay more balanced in every area of your life—it enhances your life and provides the means whereby you will feel well and happy.

5. Is anger problematic for you? What happens within you when you start to feel angry? Were either of your parents angry when you were growing up? If so, how did they model or express their anger? How do you handle other people's anger? If you find anger difficult to deal with, it is likely that this powerful emotion influences you in ways that may be destabilizing. Ask yourself if coming into harmony with this emotional energy is worth adding to your list of self-care objectives. If it is, there are numerous suggestions in subsequent chapters that may be helpful for you.

6. During the times that you are supporting others, do you feel your heart opening and taking you to a place of communion or deep compassionate connection with the people you are helping? If so, is this something that continues to inform your life experience even after work, or is it just something that occurs as part of your job?

7. Consider the gifts that you receive from helping others. Consider that you are a gift. Are you able to be the gift that keeps on giving while maintaining your health and well-being? This is the most important question.

CHAPTER

2

The Characteristics of High-Intensity Relaters

With rare exceptions, people who earn their living by helping others are drawn to their profession for two reasons—they want to help alleviate pain and suffering in the world, and they have a particular temperament that draws them to their vocation. This temperament makes them well suited for the demands of the very challenging and demanding interpersonal contexts inherent in their work.

Similarly, most people who actively and gladly choose to be caregivers in unpaid, private situations (with a family member, friend or neighbor, for example) also have the particular temperament that allows them to slide comfortably into that role.

The most prominent element of this temperament is a marked predisposition to orient to people in a uniquely empathic way. Before we begin looking at how the "helper temperament" has been defined by various theorists, we must make clear what *empathy* really means.

The *American Heritage Dictionary* defines empathy as "Identification with and understanding of another's situation, feelings, and motives; the attribution of one's own feelings to an object."[1] The *American Heritage Dictionary of Cultural Literacy* addresses the somatic component: "Identifying oneself completely with an object or person, sometimes even to the point of responding physically, as when, watching a baseball player swing at a pitch, one feels one's own muscles flex."[2]

While these descriptions of empathy are generally well understood, it is interesting to note that the word was originally associated with art appreciation. Its meaning related to one's ability to "feel into" the experience of another.[3]

The term *empathy* was introduced into popular use in the 1920s by American psychologist E.B. Titchener. He expanded on its meaning and was the first to bring the concept of empathy into the English language. Titchener believed that empathy emerges from a somatic mimicry of the distress of another, and that this mimicry generates the same feelings in oneself. This is in contrast to sympathy, which is an appreciation of someone else's difficulties but without any emotional identification with or sharing of that person's feelings.

> For our purposes, let's define *empathy* as the ability to know just what another person is feeling emotionally and somatically.

For our purposes, let's define *empathy* as the ability to know just what another person is feeling emotionally and somatically.

The "helper personality"

While the ability to relate empathically to others is an inherent human quality, those who choose to be helpers tend to relate to others in a way that sets them apart. Other theorists and I believe that this is explained by the existence of a unique helper personality.

Psychologists and other researchers have developed many ways to identify and describe the different types of personalities that individuals have. What follows is a brief discussion of the four personality constructs that help us understand the characteristics of individuals who are highly empathic—that is, who are naturally suited to the caregiving role.

Model 1: *High interpersonal intelligence*
One of the most compelling theories that supports the concept of a helper personality emerges from psychologist Howard Gardner, of the Harvard School of Education. In his 1983 book *Frames of*

Mind, Gardner deconstructs what has become the status quo consensus on what determines intelligence.

Traditionally, intelligence was understood to be a narrowly focused attribute that could be measured using an "intelligence quotient" test. The first IQ test was developed by Parisian psychologist Alfred Binet in 1900. Shortly afterward, Stanford psychologist Lewis Terman developed the first mass IQ testing for over a million new recruits during World War I. Ever since, the IQ test has been accepted as a legitimate scientific measurement tool for determining how much innate intelligence someone has.[4] The standard IQ test measures verbal and mathematical aptitudes, which are taken to be a measure of just how "smart" individuals are. Implicit in this almost universal way of thinking is that you are born with a certain IQ and that there is nothing you can do to change it. The admissions tests that most college applicants are required to take are based on this thinking, and the SATs are viewed as predictors of whether the applicant will be successful in college.

In *Frames of Mind,* Gardner refutes this notion of an inherent, narrowly defined intelligence quotient by asserting that human beings possess multiple intelligences, not just the verbal and mathematical intelligences measured by standard IQ tests. He argues that additional categories include the kinesthetic abilities of Olympic athletes and ballet dancers, the unusual musical talent of distinguished performing artists, and the "personal intelligences"—*inter*personal and *intra*personal intelligence.

Gardner believes that interpersonal intelligence is an essential feature of empathy, and he defines *interpersonal intelligence* as "the ability to understand other people: what motivates them, how they work, how to work cooperatively with them." Popular TV talk show host Oprah Winfrey exemplifies high interpersonal intelligence, which enables her to establish immediate and engaging rapport with any guest. The same is true for the popular NPR radio hosts Tom and Ray Magliozzi. Their *Car Talk* radio show, which has been broadcast since 1977, is currently one of the most downloaded podcasts from the iTunes Store's podcast directory.

Gardner argues that an individual who has high interpersonal intelligence has four distinct features:

- the ability to nurture relationships and maintain friendships
- superior leadership skills
- excellent conflict resolution abilities
- a predisposition to quickly establish rapport that is underpinned by empathy

The complement to interpersonal intelligence is *intra*personal intelligence, which Gardner defines as "a correlative ability, turned inward. It is a capacity to form an accurate, veridical model of oneself and to be able to use that model to operate effectively in life."[5] Sigmund Freud and Carl Jung exemplified what it is to have strong intrapersonal intelligence. They shared an extraordinary ability to delve into their own interior self. As a result, they developed their respective influential psychological and psychospiritual human developmental models.

As can be seen from the above, Gardner draws a clear connection between having high interpersonal intelligence and being able to relate to others empathically. His descriptions of empathy and high interpersonal intelligence both include "capacities to discern and respond appropriately to the moods, temperaments, motivations, and desires of other people." But Gardner also sees intrapersonal intelligence as an important element in what makes a person highly empathic. He states that an essential component of self-knowledge is the ability to perceive "one's own feelings and the ability to discriminate among them and draw upon them to guide behavior."[6] In other words, to have high interpersonal intelligence, a person must know, understand and act upon their own feelings as well as the feelings of others.

It is interesting to note that Gardner's theory of multiple intelligences has relevance to the way in which we raise our children. If Gardner's views were widely adopted, parents would nurture *all* of their children's strengths and natural abilities by paying close attention to how they interact with the world and how well they know themselves, rather than focusing on a culturally endorsed bias toward education that stresses excellence in cognitive-based verbal and mathematical skills. This shift in parental (and societal) attitudes would provide for greater possibilities for the support and recognition of the development of empathy, a quality that fosters human relations with greater understanding of and appreciation for our differences.

Model 2: *The Enneagram Nurturer*
The Enneagram, a well-known model for describing and differentiating personality types, evolved from Eastern mystical roots. It is now a practical and accessible model for better understanding personality that Oscar Ichazo and others have been disseminating worldwide since the early 1970s. Because the Enneagram is a modern synthesis of a number of ancient wisdom traditions, it provides a nonpathologizing model of personality that is devoid of the usual personality-disorder jargon, and it is easily understood and used by both professionals and nonprofessionals.[7]

Essentially, the Enneagram model identifies nine basic personality types that help us to understand why we behave in certain ways and our underlying motives for choosing these behaviors. Each of the nine types has its own strengths and weaknesses.[8] Although Enneagram theory asserts that each of us possesses traits of all nine personality types, it emphasizes that one of these types predominates in each individual's soul.

In my empirical research, it has become evident to me that many professional caregivers personify the Enneagram personality type Two, which is variously called the Nurturer, Giver and Caretaker. When Nurturers are at their best, they make others feel

Many professional caregivers personify the Enneagram personality type Two, which is variously called the Nurturer, Giver and Caretaker.

comfortable and welcome in their presence. They are attentive, generous, warm and highly tuned-in to the person they are relating to. Relationship is paramount in the value system of Twos—for them, there is nothing more important or personally satisfying than relating to others. They tend to be so sensitive to and perceptive about others' feelings (that is, so empathic) that they know exactly what the other person needs and instinctively respond from a place of remarkable intuitive knowingness. I've come to notice that Nurturers often know more about how another person is feeling than that other person even knows him- or herself. Natural empathy and high interpersonal intelligence are integral to the Enneagram type Two. While Nurturers are multidimensional and fit well into all kinds of environments and careers, their ability to comfortably relate to people and make friends easily gives them a natural predisposition to being in caregiving roles.

However, there is a downside or a shadow component to the Nurturer type when serving in the role as a caregiver. Enneagram Twos often have trouble asking for what they need and tend to minimize their own needs, since they are usually more comfortable giving of themselves than receiving from others. Because of their orientation to caretaking and referencing to others' needs first, it is not unusual for Nurturers to feel overburdened by people's dependence on them. Many Nurturers develop a plethora of physical symptoms as a direct result of becoming emotionally drained and energetically depleted from taking care of everybody else. Although a Two's outer presentation is often enthusiastic engagement demonstrating what appears to be a genuine interest in your problems, a surprising pattern of ongoing hidden resentment often plagues this personality type. Because Nurturers are so tuned-in to other people's feelings, it is easy for them to lose themselves in reltionships. Frequently, they harbor prohibitions to saying NO to the needs of others, and thus are prone to slipping into codependency and becoming a "no self." (This is discussed further in Chapter 7).

Over the years, having seen thousands of clients in my practice, I have noticed that it is frequently the Enneagram type Two or Nurturer who has the most problems maintaining healthy boundaries with other people. Twos are energetically so merged with the other that they typically cannot define where they end and the other person begins. When this becomes the persistent pattern in their relationships, a Two can become overly possessive and controlling, extremely needy, unhappy, and ultimately end up with soul loss (a consequence of not staying whole or maintaining appropriate boundaries with other people).

Model 3: *The highly sensitive person*
In 1996, clinical psychologist Elaine Aron published *The Highly Sensitive Person*, in which she describes a neural trait that is common in 15 to 20 percent of the population, or about fifty million Americans.[9] If that statistic is correct, then it follows that at least one or more people out of every five caregivers embodies this temperament, since highly sensitive people (HSPs) are drawn to the caregiving professions.

People who are HSPs are more easily overwhelmed when they are in a highly stimulating environment for too long. Traits common to HSPs include an awareness of subtleties in their environment, a quicker than normal startle response and a tendency to withdraw from outer stimuli such as bright lights, strong smells and loud noises. Like introverts, HSPs tend to have a rich and complex interior life that predisposes them to be deeply affected by other people's moods. This trait is similar to Gardner's intrapersonal intelligence in that HSPs tend to be unusually internally oriented and thus very sensitive to their own moods and inner perceptions. As a result, they are highly attuned to the moods and feeling states of others; thus, being empathic to what other people are experiencing comes quite naturally to them.

A person with this temperament has a nervous system that becomes more highly aroused more quickly from stimuli that other people are relatively unaffected by.[10] Consequently, HSPs tend to be more self-protective as a way to avoid getting into upsetting or overwhelming situations. While HSPs tend to be naturally more intuitive because of the way they pick up subtle energies and information that other people usually do not, their inherent heightened sensitivity predisposes them to experience what Russian physiologist Ivan Pavlov called *transmarginal inhibition*. This occurs when an individual has reached their threshold of stimulation and they become unable to cope with any more.[11] When HSPs spend too much time around other people, they can start feeling drained and depleted, just as introverts do. Feeling more in control of their environment and using strategies to conserve their vital energy are absolutely essential for caregivers who are HSPs. Often, this involves learning to say NO. (This is discussed further in Chapter 7.)

Model 4: *The intuitive empath*
It is generally true that people who are in the helping professions tend to be sensitive to the needs of others and have high degrees of empathy. Dr. Judith Orloff, a psychiatrist who uses strategies from a model she calls "energy psychiatry," teaches many of her patients to increase their awareness of their own intuitive capabilities and to become more conscious of sensing their own energy fields and the energy fields of others. Orloff has identified people who are highly sensitive *energetically* as intuitive empaths. They are very similar to both the Enneagram Nurturer and Aron's highly sensitive person.

Orloff claims that intuitive empaths give too much of their energy away to others. She describes an intuitive empath as a person

who's so sensitive that you often unknowingly absorb energy from others and are drained by it. To cope, we escape into solitude to ward off overload . . . empaths are so uncannily attuned that we feel what's going on inside other people emotionally and physically, making it hard to distinguish whether it's us or them. We get struck down, and don't know what hit us.[12]

Orloff calls intuition "the language of energy":

Intuition brings magic to traditional wellness approaches, but also opens into the intriguing realm of energy fields—realms that radiate from people, places, clients, the night sky.[13]

She goes on to explain that we know things intuitively through myriad perceptual cues or what she calls "vibes." "People and situations can give off welcoming positive energy that invigorates, or oppressive negative energy that repels."[14] Some intuitive empaths feel a pit in their stomach that leaves them nauseous and instantly enervated when they are around people who are negative. The same people feel a sense of expansion, warmth and well-being when they are around people who are happy, generous and compassionate.

In fact, these different "intuitive knowings" are instantly sensed and felt by us all. They are part of the primitive and instinctual early warning system that provides us with need-to-know, instantaneous information that bypasses our more evolved rationally based prefrontal cortex. How do you know if someone is emanating negative energy? Orloff lists a number of ways in which an average person experiences being in the presence of someone who is emanating negative energy:

You experience the sense of being demeaned, constricted or attacked. You intuitively feel unsafe, tense, or on guard. You sense prickly, off putting vibes. You can't wait to get away from them. Your energy starts to fizzle. You feel beleaguered or ill.[15]

Orloff insists that in order to maintain good physical and emotional health, it is essential to know whether you are an intuitive empath.

The risks of being highly empathic

Individuals who identify with one or more of the character traits or predispositions inherent in these descriptions of the helper temperament generally have a heightened sensitivity to their environment and other people. They are also more likely than others to take in and absorb the vibes (energy) they feel emanating from the people around them.

For example, a deeply empathic client of mine, Anna, was attending to the palliative care needs of a dying friend. Anna asked me for help because after leaving her friend, Anna felt a constriction in her throat and tightness in her chest, and her arms stayed numb for hours afterward. We confirmed through muscle testing that Anna had no energetic boundaries with her friend's dying process—she was absorbing her friend's anguish about dying and leaving her husband and two young children. Anna felt she could no longer be around her dying friend because her energetic boundaries were too porous. In other words, Anna was unable to shield herself because she felt too deeply into her friend's deep sadness and despair. Anna, like so many other intuitive empaths that I work with, was absorbing her friend's energy of hovering or imminent death right into her own body, a process called somatization.

Another client, Sheila, seems to have highly sensitive radar for anyone who is angry. When she picks up these anger vibes, Sheila immediately feels her throat and jaw get tight. In her own words, she feels her "entire energy body contract" around her. Sometimes it feels as though she is suddenly in the grips of a stifling bear hug, with powerful arms tightly pressing in around her.

It is important to note that highly empathic people are also sensitive to the positive energy of the people around them. They are likely the first ones to detect, for example, that an apology is authentic and sincere—they are able to effortlessly discriminate between someone who is sincere and someone who is being manipulative in order to exploit or take advantage of them.

Empaths may also absorb energy from people who are experiencing traumatic global and collective events (such as wars, natural disasters and the overthrow of a repressive regime) that are occurring halfway around the world.

As I describe in *Dynamic Energetic Healing®*, highly empathic people are characterized as frequently having very poor *energetic boundaries*. Individuals who are intuitive empaths also have an energetic tendency to somaticize—that is, to unconsciously process all of this stress-filled information through their physical bodies. This is what's happening to Anna when she feels her throat and chest tighten after visits with her dying friend. Indeed, all individuals who are highly empathic, and thus more likely to become "infected" by the energy of others, are at increased risk of having their well-being compromised. In other words, they are even more likely than other high-intensity relaters to experience burnout, vicarious and secondary traumatization, compassion fatigue and psychotoxic contamination (all of which are described in Chapter 1).

> As I describe in *Dynamic Energetic Healing®*, highly empathic people are characterized as frequently having very poor energetic boundaries.

But there is hope. All high-intensity relaters can learn to use intentional and effective strategies to protect themselves when in the role of caregiver. Chapters 5 through 12 of this book outline a wide variety of actions that you can implement to take better care of yourself—to protect yourself more effectively from the negative energy you are absorbing from the people around you. As you'll see, the most important elements in many of these strategies are the need to acknowledge what's true about yourself and to accept your own degree of sensitivity.

Before I present the practical strategies high-intensity relaters can use to cope with the myriad challenges they face every day, I need to discuss another huge challenge that all caregivers face—the woeful lack of support that we receive from our society in general. This is a difficult issue for many caregivers, who may feel isolated and abandoned. You care for and spend time supporting others, but who supports you? Like many others, you may not have a partner who is able or willing to support you, or a network of understanding friends. Despite this, there is compelling experimental evidence that there are sources of support for caregivers that you may not be aware of—the power of your mind and the power of humanity's collective mind. Also available to you are various transpersonal resources. These are referred to in religious literature, but in rather mysterious terms that don't always make clear how to access and apply these resources. Some of the evidence for the power of these internal and transpersonal resources is summarized in Chapter 4. However, I feel it is important to first highlight societal pressures that can prevent many caregivers and helpers from getting the support that they need in order to stay healthy. The next chapter discusses some of these issues, which include current economic influences and some big-impact noneconomic issues that touch all of our lives.

Questions and Exercises

1. Because of their exceptional levels of sensitivity, many high-intensity relaters tend to avoid conflict by accommodating to the needs of others. Is this at all true for you? If so, why? Does this make your life easier or harder? In addition, Enneagram

Twos tend to be pleasers; their shadow side is to not ask for what they need for themselves, which often leads to them becoming resentful. Where do you see yourself fitting in here?

2. Do you honestly express your needs to your partner, parents, children, friends and those you are helping? Do you minimize your needs instead? If so, why?

3. What are your tendencies in your helping relationships? Do you feel everything in your body and use that information knowingly? Or do you internalize your clients' fears and stresses, generating chronic physical symptoms in yourself? Are you the same way in your personal relationships? Or are you better insulated emotionally in your relationships with family, friends and colleagues?

4. Do you know what Enneagram number you are? If not, check out Baron and Wagele's book, *The Enneagram Made Easy; Discover the 9 Types of People.*[16]

5. Would you consider yourself among the 15 to 20 percent of the general population that possess the neural trait Elaine Aron calls the Highly Sensitive Person? If so, what do you do to ensure proper self-care in order to maintain emotional balance and not become overwhelmed?

6. Do you feel others' vibes and tend to absorb energy from others, often ending up feeling sickened and depleted from those encounters? Have you ever explored "subtle energies" to learn more about how this happens? However you refer to them, the feelings or energies that emanate from other people and environments can profoundly affect you. Some people are more sensitive to these energies, which the Chinese medical model calls *chi*, the subtle energy that composes all things in

the universe (not just in humans). How would you rate your sensitivity to picking up and reading these subtle energies? If you are sensitive to them, do you feel it comes with the territory of being a high-intensity relater?

3

Our Society Creates Extra Challenges for High-Intensity Relaters

One thing I am sure we can all agree on is that you need good physical and mental energy in order to accomplish anything important. It requires good stamina to get up and go to work every day to earn a living, do the shopping, be an involved parent, and have additional time on the side to exercise and make love.

As a resident of this twenty-first century, my perception that the demands placed on us are relentless and increasingly overwhelming is constantly being reinforced. It is reported by various sources that the majority of medical complaints today are stress induced. Roughly three quarters of Americans experience stress-related symptoms that compel them to seek medical help. These include physical symptoms (77%) and psychological symptoms (73%). Additionally, almost half of Americans (48%) believe that their stress has increased over the past five years (as of 2007). Physical symptoms include fatigue (51%), headaches (44%), digestive malaise (34%), muscle tension (30%) and changes in appetite (23%). Psychological effects of stress include experiencing irritability or frequent anger (50%) [including the proclivity of 54% of Americans to argue with people close to them], general feelings of nervousness (45%),

> In this twenty-first century, the demands placed on us are relentless and increasingly overwhelming.

depletion of energy and exhaustion (45%) and mood swings or feeling more prone to cry (35%). In addition, insomnia is on the rise—48% of Americans report lying awake at night due to stress.[1] These statistics are troubling in and of themselves, but when one considers that high-intensity relaters may be even more prone to these stress-related maladies than other individuals, the seriousness of the situation becomes undeniable.

Unfortunately, Western society as a whole does little to offset these relentless pressures and demands. In this chapter, I focus on four particular aspects of modern Western society that put pressure on everyone—including caregivers—and make the caregiving role more challenging.

Current economic pressures

As of the writing of this book in March of 2011, our country is in the throes of a recession worse than anything experienced for decades. With the official national unemployment rates just below 10 percent and nearly seven million Americans currently out of work, enormous stresses are placed on people who lose their jobs and their homes. In September of 2010, home foreclosures were at near record levels. "More than 2.3 million homes have been repossessed by lenders since the recession began in December 2007, according to RealtyTrac. The firm estimates more than 1 million American households are likely to lose their homes to foreclosure during 2010."[2] Over seven million borrowers, accounting for about 12 percent of all the households with a mortgage, had either missed payments or were in foreclosure as of March 2010, according to Lender Processing Services.[3] These stresses and economic traumas are passed on to the people who are doing everything they can to support the individuals and families who are directly affected by the economic downturn. For example, people who work in human resources agencies are coping with trying to help more clients who are in extreme need of support and assistance, while at the same time state and federal govern-ments continue to reduce their funding and eliminate many of their jobs.

Current noneconomic pressures

There are also serious noneconomic traumas threatening large numbers of people today. Ten years ago there were approximately 500,000 Americans diagnosed with Alzheimer's disease. That number is now over five million. According to a report issued by the Alzheimer's Association in March 2011, "Nearly 15 million unpaid caregivers help someone with Alzheimer's and other forms of dementia in the United States—37 percent more than last year." William Thies, chief medical and scientific officer of the Alzheimer's Association has reported that Alzheimer's "is the sixth-leading cause of death in the country, and the only one among the top 10 that has no prevention or cure." This creates enormous strain on families who are frequently left with the burden of taking care of their loved one who is afflicted by this disease. Cur-rent statistics indicate that family members "provide 17 billion hours of unpaid care, valued at $202.6 billion."[4] This situation is expected to get worse before it gets better. Unless a cure is found in the very near future, by the time the baby boomers reach their late sixties and early seventies, one out of every eight of them will be afflicted by this horrible and ravaging disease. New statistics suggest that someone in the United States develops the disease every sixty-nine seconds.[5] Professionals and the adult children who become the caregivers of individuals affected by Alzheimer's are going to be overwhelmed by the demands placed on them to care for and financially support this growing population of dis-abled individuals. This will soon become a collective trauma of massive proportions.

I would like to focus on one source of noneconomic pressure in particular—post-traumatic stress disorder (PTSD). As I stated in my first book,[6] many clients who are diagnosed by a physician as having anxiety or depression are, in fact, suffering from the long-term undiagnosed effects of post-traumatic stress disorder.

PTSD occurs when an individual has been exposed to an overwhelming life experience that creates long-term deleterious consequences. The consequences or symptoms of this disorder vary from person to person, but what is emblematic of PTSD is its duration. If the specific stress symptoms following an overwhelming trauma persist for more than six months, without adequate treatment the symptoms frequently go on for years, become chronic, and significantly impair and interfere with the person's life. Symptoms include flashbacks, night terrors, dissociation, extreme depression and anxiety, disproportionate anger and rage, toxic shame, self-medication leading to drug addiction and alcoholism, self-isolation, and the inability to maintain relationships. Additionally, it's common for somatic complaints to become chronic physical symptoms and disease processes such as irritable bowel syndrome, fibromyalgia, musculoskeletal problems and migraine headaches. I believe that PTSD is probably the most underreported and misdiagnosed serious mental health disorder, largely due to the fact that many clinicians haven't been trained to identify the multifaceted symptom complex of PTSD, and that they are ill-equipped and untrained to treat it capably.

> Professionals and the adult children who become the caregivers of individuals affected by Alzheimer's are going to be overwhelmed by the demands placed on them.

With such a high proportion of Americans losing their livelihoods and their homes, millions of Americans are now the "walking wounded" who have PTSD, whether they know it or not. They, along with those traumatized by dysfunctional families and specific childhood events, constitute an entire subculture of Americans suffering from the long-term effects of multiple loss. Added to their numbers are what the Pentagon has recently identified as approximately 20 percent of returning veterans from Iraq and Afghanistan (about 300,000) who are suffering from PTSD, and the inordinate number of veterans who return suffering from traumatic brain injuries.

Post-traumatic stress disorder exponentially increases the challenges faced by caregivers and helpers. An increasing proportion of those you are helping have undoubtedly suffered from long-term financial stress, and/or the after-effects of childhood emotional or sexual abuse, and/or are currently being haunted by the ghosts and demons of horrific battle memories. The natural tendency of these PTSD sufferers is to deny and minimize the overwhelming life experiences that are at the root of their flashbacks, their inability to be with other people, their disproportionate anger and rage toward their loved ones, or their use of drugs and alcohol as a way to seek temporary solace from the horrors within.

> Millions of Americans are now the "walking wounded" who have PTSD, whether they know it or not.

Let us not be naïve. Caring for someone who has PTSD poses particular—and quite daunting—challenges. Those who are suffering with this kind of emotional pain tend to carry information fields within them that are laden with psychotoxic energy. Often, although these clients know they need help, they are so frightened and well defended that they are unable to allow a caregiver to revisit with them the dark places that they are trying so desperately to avoid.

Compounding the challenge for you as a caregiver is the fact that you may not be adequately trained to help those who are afflicted by PTSD. It is also worth considering that you may be struggling to cope with the after-effects of a significant trauma in your own past. If you are, your interactions with clients may restimulate and exacerbate your own PTSD symptoms. This occurs via the process of negative countertransference, which is discussed in my first book, *Dynamic Energetic Healing*®.

The limitations of allopathic medicine

An important question to consider is how our current medical model is helping us to stay healthy. The medical system that we in the Western world are accustomed to using is by and large called *allopathic* medicine. Allopathic medicine is defined as "a method of treating disease with remedies that produce effects different from those caused by the disease itself."[7] This is the healthcare system that we are paying higher and higher insurance premiums for.

Allopathic medicine is an important approach for "treating disease" that has already taken hold in a person, and for addressing acute care issues through surgical intervention. However, it does not make preventative care a priority, and it is increasingly relying on pharmaceutical drugs as the answer for most of our medical problems.

A good example of this trend is the change in how psychiatrists treat patients. Since the proliferation of pharmaceutical drugs for treating common psychiatric disorders such as depression and anxiety began in the mid-1950s, the way in which psychiatrists interact with their patients has changed dramatically. On average, psychiatrists now spend fifteen minutes with their patients to inquire about their symptoms and modify or renew their prescriptions of pharmaceutical drugs for their treatment. It is now widely acknowledged in the psychiatric literature that most psychiatrists don't have the time to have meaningful discussions with their patients in order to provide substantive psychotherapy.

You may be struggling to cope with the after-effects of a significant trauma in your own past.

While the medications prescribed for depression and anxiety can be helpful, they generally don't resolve the underlying issues that generate the symptoms. Instead, the drugs are designed to reduce the person's extreme highs and lows—their symptoms—by modifying their brain chemistry so the person can get through each day and get back to work. Insurance companies pay for these visits because they are considered "medically necessary" to "stabilize" the patient. That's not necessarily a bad thing, but many people report that medication alone doesn't make their symptoms go away completely.

I know of three colleagues who have been taking antidepressant medications prescribed by their doctor for years. The symptoms that they initially came in for persist, albeit at a lower level than before they began taking their medication. Their doctor tells them that their depression is being "well managed," and thus there's no need to do anything else.

I don't mean to criticize medical doctors in general—I recognize that most are hard-working and very dedicated. But because of the underlying Western medical paradigm at the foundation of their approach, and the restrictions imposed by managed care health insurance, Western medicine falls far short of providing the support and ancillary care that helpers and caregivers require. Thus, one of the major premises of this book is that relying on the pharmaceuticals used in traditional Western medicine is not the best approach for high-intensity relaters who need better ways to take care of themselves.

In stark contrast to traditional Western medicine is an alternative known as complementary and alternative medical approaches (CAM). CAM is a group of diverse medical and healthcare systems and practices

> Western medicine falls far short of providing the support and ancillary care that helpers and caregivers require.

that are not generally considered part of conventional Western medicine, including such practices as yoga, meditation, biofeedback, working with a naturopath or chiropractor, guided imagery and traditional Chinese medicine such as acupuncture. Statistics show that Americans are turning to these CAM practices more and more to meet specific healthcare needs that the Western medical paradigm is unable to address sufficiently.

According to the 2007 National Health Interview Survey (NHIS), approximately 38 percent of adults in the United States are using some form of CAM.[8] These statistics show that Americans are beginning to catch on to the worldwide trend that favors alternative medicine over traditional Western medicine.

> In 1991 Americans made more visits to unconventional health care providers (425 million) than to conventional doctors (388 million). . . . Worldwide, only ten to thirty percent of people use conventional medicine, 70 to 90 percent use alternative medicine.[9]

I strongly believe that most people want to take personal responsibility for doing whatever they can to feel better when they are hurting or in pain, and these statistics indicate that many are turning to CAM approaches to help them do that. Granted, agreeing to fill your family physician's prescription for pills that will relieve your stress-related insomnia and panic attacks is taking some kind of personal responsibility. But many people are discovering that CAM provides healthier and even better options, even though they may require more time and effort than simply taking a pill.

> Americans are beginning to catch on to the worldwide trend that favors alternative medicine over traditional Western medicine.

While many people are still loathe to consider many of these alternative or complementary practices, the statistics cited above indicate that increasing numbers of people are willing to take more personal responsibility in order to take better care of themselves.

The role of the media

In ancient Greece, dating as far back as 1400 B.C.E., the famous Oracle of Delphi was consulted by peasants and farmers who wanted guidance on planting and harvesting, and by prominent leaders such as Sophocles and Alexander the Great. People came from all over Greece and the rest of Europe to have their questions answered by the Pythia, the priestess of Apollo. For over fourteen centuries, this role was filled by women who were the mediums through which the god Apollo spoke. From its temple on Mount Parnassus, the Oracle of Delphi disseminated prophecies and information that shaped historical outcomes by determining military and political tactics. Such was the importance of the Oracle of Delphi that the ancients believed it to be the center (*omphalos*) of the world.[10]

Today, we live in the digital age, in which technology sends us a constant stream of information and delivers data instantly. We actively seek some of this information. But instead of having to make an arduous journey to a distant place to get it, we have the internet search engine known as Google. In our family, when a question emerges during a discussion and no one knows the answer, we jokingly remind each other to consult "the oracle." Within seconds of typing an inquiry into the Google bar on the computer, we are confronted with hundreds of related links directing us to the information that we desire. Human beings are curious creatures and are always open to new experiences. Whether it's a science-based question about the long-term health of Alaskan fisheries, the six-month weather patterns that will affect next season's wheat and rye planting, or the best way to make a flaky pie crust, the oracle can be easily consulted to provide a plethora of useful data. In our information age the desire to acquire and have access to "need-to-know" information has taken on a life of its own. The availability and accessibility of information can make our lives easier on many levels.

At the same time, we also contribute to "the information tsunami"—it is not just a one-way channel through which we are inundated. More and more people are spending a significant amount of their time communicating through e-mail, Facebook and other forms of social networking. While much of this is required for one's job, the inherent seduction embedded in e-mail, for example, with links to internet articles and YouTube videos, can often become a significant time sink and major distraction from one's intended work.

Not all of the information that influences us is intentionally sought. The shadow side of our evolving interconnected digital world is that we are constantly being bombarded by information in many different and insidious forms. This inundation of information is, essentially, like any other form of pollution—we contribute to it, we get contaminated by it, and it has profound consequences for us personally and collectively. The penetrating impact of these various information contaminants is not widely understood and, except for advertisers, political strategists and public relations firms, most people grossly underestimate its impact on our lives and our spirits.

> This inundation of information is, essentially, like any other form of pollution.

How the media overwhelm and create fear

The most pernicious effect of media pollution on our lives is that it influences us energetically. Being exposed to continual information about the increasing violence that people inflict on others and on the earth fosters feelings of hopelessness, overwhelm and, perhaps most importantly, a profound feeling of a general lack of safety.

The purpose of the one-way media channels (through which we receive information from television, newspapers, online news sites, and so on) is to report on the latest terrorist threat, a local serial killer, the devastating effects of changing weather patterns and powerful destructive storms, and the growing state and national deficits that can threaten your job and retirement savings. The results can be overwhelming for viewers and listeners.

When we saw jets colliding with the World Trade Center towers over and over, and bodies floating in the floodwaters of New Orleans while people who were stuck on their rooftops waited to be rescued, the media became the focus of everyone's attention. Because these horrific images were shown constantly, the capriciousness of life illustrated by these events continued to traumatize our nation.

The intended purpose of the two-way media channels (social networking, chat lists, online forums, and so on) is to facilitate communication between people in a positive way. But do these channels really do that? Many people argue that interactive media provide easy access for individuals to reach out to and interact with people they otherwise would not. But while the relative anonymity of interacting with a user name behind a screen emboldens some, the context is one that provides protection from true and authentic emotional intimacy. After all, if things become emotionally challenging, it takes only a tap on a keyboard to immediately dismiss yourself from interacting with the other person.

No one is immune from media overwhelm. The vast network of information that is constantly available has us mesmerized.

The media as our first reference point

As the many sources of information continue to become digitized, the media in all their various forms are becoming the substitute for what religious and spiritual practices have always brought us— namely, the feeling of being connected to something greater than ourselves. Additionally, as people

> No one is immune from media overwhelm.

become more tethered to their digital devices and screens, their human tendency to be self-referential becomes more and more a thing of the past. "The screen's the thing" as that external reference point continues to demand more and more of our attention.

Knowledge is becoming something "out there," and inquiry into our interior self is being progressively marginalized. For most of us, the electronic media are the vehicles through which we experience vicarious connection to all things larger and greater than ourselves, as we each yearn to heal our fundamental sense of aloneness in the universe. Some refer to this as our "core soul wound." We're like the drones who constitute the Borg collective in *Star Trek*, except that we experience the "sounds of the billions of voices of the collective" through the media. Global wireless communication and the web are bringing this reality closer to each of us every day. Our growing connection to the media is our unconscious attempt to heal our core soul wound of feeling separate and alone.

The Dreaming Media

Therein lies the power of the media's seductive grip on each of us. As this outward focus becomes more deeply embedded as the zeitgeist of our culture, awareness of the need for structured, daily and conscious self-care is being overrun and usurped by what I call the Dreaming Media. The Dreaming Media is like a dark, collective spirit that we are becoming more and more closely related to. The digital world is everywhere and its insidious influence continues to grow day by day. We are gradually losing our sense of individuality thanks to our seemingly omnipresent connection with the media—we've become more influenced by the information we receive through the one-way and two-way channels of media communication than by the self-reflective inner states of awareness that are the cornerstone of self-care. The constant barrage of information we are subjected to reduces our ability to know what's really true of and for ourselves, and diminishes our sense of personal autonomy. Thus, we become even more easily influenced

> The Dreaming Media is like a dark, collective spirit that we are becoming more and more closely related to.

by the Dreaming Media as we shift our focus to digital interconnectedness rather than on maintaining a strong inner connection with ourselves. The digital world has become *our* world—in a sense, it has become our lifeline.

I have conceived of the Dreaming Media as a new and emerging archetype. Swiss psychologist Carl Jung popularized the concepts of archetypes and the collective unconscious. A brief tutorial is in order.

According to Jung, the collective unconscious is the ancient "shared wisdoms" and experiences that connect all human beings with respect to how we encounter and experience our personal existence as humans. Jung found that archetypal patterns and images appear in every culture and in every time period of human history. An archetype is an ancient *shared image or symbol* that represents an energy or a human experience that is necessary for people to experience life in its completeness. Familiar examples include Mother-Father, Warrior, Athlete, Prophet, Judge, Thief, and Lover-Beloved. These archetypal figures have been portrayed in fairy tales, myths, and creation stories in every culture, and can even be seen in the cave paintings of preindustrial indigenous societies. To account for the fact that the archetypes behave according to the same laws in all cases, Jung suggested that we are all linked through our collective unconscious mind, and thus we share what he called a single Universal Unconscious.

My concept of the Dreaming Media as a new and emerging archetype meets all but one of the criteria of Jung's classical definition of *archetype* (namely, the Dreaming Media isn't ancient). Due to the pervasive and growing international influence of the Dreaming Media archetype, it structures our imagination and is distinctly human. It shapes matter (nature) as well as mind or psyche. After all, as our society becomes increasingly digitized, the physical nature of our reality is changing. Think about computers on every desk, televisions in almost every household, and cell phones being transformed into smart phones carried by more people every day. Entire cities are now becoming one big Wi-Fi hotspot.

The Dreaming Media is cross-cultural and recognized by everyone throughout the world. A recent article in The *New York Times* about the proliferation of cell phones in India points out that

> India's nearly 400 million cell phone users still account for only a third of the population. But the technology has seeped down the social strata, into slums and small towns and villages, becoming that rare Indian possession to traverse the walls of caste and region and class; a majority of subscribers are now outside the major cities and wealthiest states. And while the average bill, of less than $5 per month, represents 7 percent of the average Indian's income, enough Indians apparently consider the sacrifice worth it: if present trends continue, in five years every Indian will have a cell phone.[11]

This is in a developing country where more people have access to a cell phone than to a clean toilet! As a by-product of technology, the Dreaming Media is playing an essential role in the creation of the world and the human mind itself. It is determining how people interact with one another and is quickly becoming our primary link to the human collective.

As these global information fields are being channeled into our personal energy fields through the various forms of technology, this new archetype is essentially *dreaming our current reality*. What I mean is that people are losing their volition to *consciously* choose how best to deeply take care of themselves because of the ubiquitous distraction of the media messages that draw them into participating in the larger collective fields of information. This is in spite of the illusion that technology generates more choices for us. The Dreaming Media has become so powerful that it has taken on a life of its own, and we are all in danger of being assimilated by it.

Of course I'm not referring to just cell phones here. Let's consider television. Presently, 99 percent of American households have at least one television, and 66 percent have three or more TVs. The average U.S. home has 2.24 televisions,[12] and the TV is on for more than six hours per day. And while we're not quite to the point of burning books and replacing them with larger and larger TV screens as in Ray Bradbury's *Fahrenheit 451*, television screens are becoming larger and less expensive, 3D televisions are beginning to take hold in the market, and television viewing is now merging with the internet through streaming content and video gaming.

While the information tsunami continues to barrel its way through nearly every household via the omnipresent television(s), the complex, visually enticing virtual worlds being created by game developers are also proliferating—another indication of how the Dreaming Media archetype is structuring our distinctly human imaginations. The popularity of these games continues to grow, and online players are now linked to the human collective on a global scale as they create connections with people all over the world. To give one example, the Blizzard game development company introduced World of Warcraft six years ago. Currently, the game's more than twelve million subscribers live in North America, Europe, China, Korea, Australia, New Zealand, Singapore, Thailand, Malaysia, Indonesia, the Philippines, Chile, Argentina, Taiwan and Macau.[13] Future growth is expected to continue thanks to Blizzard launching expansion packs every year.

On the face of it, the increasing prevalence of online games sounds potentially positive. Online gaming may be "shaping matter" to create a "new human"—one who is merged with technology in a way that helps people from all nationalities interact. This new human may be a harbinger of a new and emerging human consciousness. Yet I wonder—is online gaming fostering greater interconnectedness in a way that supports our personal growth and development, spiritual evolution and well-being? Or is it some form of soul stealing? What will this new human be like?

Theorists believe that our personal shadows (that is, our disavowed emotions such as our strong, primitive sexual and violent impulses) get split off from us as individuals into the collective unconscious. This collective unconscious carries billions of people's individual shadow parts to form a collective cloud of dark, marginalized emotional material. The Dreaming Media is so pernicious because it channels this dark emotional material back to us in the form of increasingly sexual, gross, violent and in-your-face special effects. These sounds and images juice up our sympathetic nervous systems to demand our attention, creating a perpetual fight-or-flight response.

Why are increasingly "realistic" first-person combat video games among the most popular bestsellers worldwide? Because we are drawn to the sensationalized media expressions of the parts of ourselves we have excluded and split off. We unconsciously seek out our missing parts—which are vividly portrayed through the media—to try to heal and reintegrate these lost parts into our selves. They are "out there" on the screen so we can vicariously experience the marginalized parts of us. We are drawn to these rejected parts of our inner selves so strongly that we become addicted to the media that reflect them. Until we each recognize this split within ourselves and decide to work on integrating our lost and rejected parts, we can look forward to more and more intensification of these various aspects of the Dreaming Media.

Media and addiction

The emerging Dreaming Media archetype does not discriminate. Caregivers and helpers are under enormous pressures and stress, and the various media provide a quick and accessible escape from the stresses during and after the workday. However, although I enjoy watching a well-made movie as much as many others do, I consciously do not allow the internet (or television) to dominate my free time every night after work. Based on my own experience, I know that if I overindulge in using electronic media my life-force energy becomes depleted and I become seduced away from staying focused on my important self-care regimen, such as spending time talking with my family, reading and practicing regular meditation.

Perhaps watching television nightly is your way of winding down and relaxing after a day of caring for others, but does it contribute to your efforts to stay emotionally and physically balanced, or does it hinder them? Are you aware that staying "plugged in" to the media has the potential to become addicting, and that you may someday discover that you just cannot do without it? Being addicted to the process of interacting with the media in its many and varied forms is becoming all too common. The therapeutic community is seeing more overt signs of addiction to various forms of media in adolescents and young adults in particular. In fact, there is considerable discussion within the American Psychiatric Association of whether to add *internet addiction* to the next edition of its *Diagnostic and Statistical Manual of Mental Disorders*. Mental health professionals are seeing this growing trend throughout the country and beginning to take it quite seriously.

Media addiction can happen to anyone and be related to any or all varieties of the Dreaming Media, including surfing the internet, watching television, or watching video-on-demand that gets streamed to your television or computer. Computers and smart phones provide all kinds of entertainment and distraction. Their sensationalized, eye-grabbing multimedia seductiveness can have the same effect on people as Dr. Timothy Leary's 1960s exhortations to "turn on, tune in, drop out." The major theme of Leary's message related to LSD as a way to expand one's consciousness. Today, with the impact of the information tsunami, we are being exhorted by the marketers and advertisers (wherever we look or listen) to *turn on* our digital device of choice, *tune in* to the media that grab our attention, and *drop out* of our relationship to external reality and leave all our troubles behind. This media trance is just as addictive and self-destructive as any other kind of addiction.

It might be reasonably argued that the issue of media addiction is more relevant to those people who grew up in the digital age from the early 1990s to the present time. But the baby boomers, many of whom are entering their 60s now, are just as vulnerable to the seductions generated by the Dreaming Media.

George

For example, a client in his mid-50s, George, had managed to overcome his alcohol addiction after several months of focused therapy. He lived by himself and enjoyed reading, but while surfing the internet he discovered the World of Warcraft online game mentioned earlier. George had never played an online game before, but it wasn't long before he was spending many hours every day playing the game late into the night. He didn't mention it to me until a couple of months after he began playing. He waxed enthusiastic about the amazing graphics and the depth of interaction he was experiencing with people from all over the world. But when George's sleep became compromised and his performance at work started to get the wrong kind of attention, we soon uncovered that his involvement with the game was a substitute for his previous addiction to alcohol. He had unwittingly discovered a replacement for a self-medicating tool that was ultimately just as self-destructive as alcohol abuse had been. It took George some time to fully realize the depth of the game's hold on him, but eventually he was able to relinquish his powerful desire to sign on and immerse himself in the addictive virtual world.

George is an example of someone who struggles with addiction issues. Like anyone else, caregivers and helpers can easily become addicted to media stimulation. In fact, they may discover that constant overstimulation leads them to the point at which their nervous systems begin to crave even more media stimulation. Is this not similar to our culture's addiction to caffeine, the chemical in coffee, tea and Coke that is the fuel that keeps the engines of industry going?

The relevance of these societal factors to high-intensity relaters

Trauma has been described as an overwhelming life experience. The economic and noneconomic forms of loss-related traumas currently being experienced by millions of people are unprecedented in our nation's recent history. While I hope that the indicators and predictions for the future are wrong, I believe there is a great likelihood that the global recession will expand and worsen before there is a leveling off. Unfortunately, our allopathic medical system is not geared to help people cope with these traumas in effective ways. In addition, record numbers of individuals are struggling with post-traumatic stress disorder—whether they realize it or not—yet most caregivers have little or no training in how to help someone with this debilitating disorder. Meanwhile, the Dreaming Media is becoming more and more demanding of our time, energy, and attention.

Moderation is always recommended, and yet staying highly stimulated to accomplish more is often regarded as virtuous in our society. But consider that the nervous systems of high-intensity relaters are already highly stimulated from the demands of their work. The information tsunami that barrels through the Dreaming Media demands more and more time, energy, and attention from us all, which puts caregivers in danger of reaching their overstimulation threshold much more quickly. High-intensity relaters generally need soft music and restful self-care

> High-intensity relaters generally need soft music and restful self-care practices in place of coming home to virtual battlefields and intense action movies on a nightly basis.

practices in place of coming home to virtual battlefields and intense action movies on a nightly basis. Balance is always preferred. As a high-intensity relater, how do you characterize your relationship to the Dreaming Media?

How is one to take care of oneself amid increasing family, national, and global trauma and stress, and in the face of the relentless information tsunami? This question is particularly relevant to the times we are living in. With so many worries, responsibilities and demands pressing on you as a caregiver, the need for you to care for and replenish yourself appears more urgent than ever before.

> As a high-intensity relater, how do you characterize your relationship to the Dreaming Media?

The challenges I have discussed in this chapter seem so large and amorphous at times that they often generate feelings of overwhelm about our capacity to stay in control of our lives. This experience of overwhelm is frequently the underlying reason that people seek help—their normal coping abilities have been overrun and their ability to maintain homeostasis has been compromised. While the media provokes much of this, it can also provide temporary balm to the increasing global fears of financial, political and macroeconomic uncertainty through distraction and trance-inducing high-tech entertainment. Yet when the screen is turned off, the internal apprehensions still persist.

So many of these challenges seem to be imposing themselves on us from the outside, but the next chapter prompts you to consider how your thinking can create positive self-care changes from the inside. Chapter 4 asks you to consider paradigms that may be new to you in order to reassess your current ways of thinking about how the world works and makes sense. Consider that you have the resources within you to combat these multitudinous challenges and to actually shift your inner "assemblage point" to adjust to shifting realities and maintain self-coherence and well-being. Read on.

Questions and Exercises

1. Does anyone in your extended family suffer with Alzheimer's disease? If so, are you able to offer support to them while still taking care of yourself?

2. Do you use any CAM practices regularly? To what degree do they support you as a caregiver or helper? Do they make a noticeable difference in how you feel and function in your job?

3. Take some time to define your relationship with the media. How much of your interaction with the media is necessary for work, and how much is for recreational pursuits? Does the time that you spend voluntarily with various forms of media interfere with pursuing your additional responsibilities and interests? Good ongoing self-care requires commitment and the time necessary to do the things you determine are important to keep your life moving in a positive direction. Decide if your relationship with media detract from or help you to accomplish your self-care goals.

4. As a caregiver or helper, what do you need to replenish your stores of vital energy at the end of each workday? After giving out energy to others all day, how do you structure your evenings to enable you to sleep well and wake up refreshed the next morning? Do you use some form of media to unwind and de-stress? If so, is your nervous system sufficiently calmed y the time you turn in for the night?

5. List your three favorite media sources. Do you feel an addictive pull from any of them? Do you have more than one e-mail or social media account? In your discretionary time, do any of these keep pulling you back for "just five more minutes"? If

so, reflect on your self-care goals to decide whether your relationship with the media is interfering in any way. Decide what, if any, changes you need to make happen. Use the media for your benefit—don't allow the media to use you.

6. Does your discretionary use of the media help you to feel more connected to others, or does it tend to isolate you?

7. What are your sources of news? Does staying current with the news help you feel more secure knowing about what's going on in the world? Or do you end up feeling more agitated and apprehensive? If staying current generates anxiety, consider modifying your relationship to the media to help you maintain a positive mental attitude about your life, the planet and other people.

CHAPTER

4

Evidence of the Power
of Your Mind

We've talked about how difficult it is for caregivers to protect themselves from burnout and compassion fatigue. We've also talked about how Western society and medicine do not provide adequate support for high-intensity relaters. But there are some exciting new developments that point to how you can use the power of your mind to take care of yourself, and to use nonphysical approaches to help other people heal.

This chapter provides a brief discussion of the new language and concepts that are emerging from the exciting interface of cutting-edge scientific discoveries with ancient spiritual knowledge. When used properly and consistently, these approaches will not just reduce but eliminate some of the hazards of caregiving, such as burnout, compassion fatigue, and absorbing the pain and trauma of others. What follows is a fascinating journey into how your words, thoughts and intentions can have a profoundly healing effect on those with whom you are interacting, and how you can use the abilities of your mind to maintain your own self-care and heal yourself as well.

Dr. Larry Dossey has been researching and writing about the effects of our thoughts, attitudes and consciousness in our relationship with all living things (as well as inanimate objects) for well over a decade. Having trained as a Western medical doctor, his interest

> When used properly and consistently, these approaches cannot just reduce but eliminate some of the hazards of caregiving.

in complementary healing has propelled him into the forefront of some very exciting original research reflecting the direction in which Western medicine is evolving. In his book *Reinventing Medicine: Beyond Mind-Body to a New Era of Healing*, he has summarized the evolution of Western medicine by dividing it into three primary eras. While most people have come to accept the value of having a broken bone set with the help of an X-ray, the healing power of our thoughts affecting others is often questioned.

Era I and Era II medicine

In Era I medicine, treatments that most of us are familiar with dominated Western medical applications. Era I began near the end of the nineteenth century with the adoption of the so-called germ theory of disease. The treatment protocols of this phase came out of medical research, and they focus on the concrete and mechanistic workings of the physical body. These approaches include surgery, pharmaceutical drugs, radiation and X-rays, taking biopsies of tissue samples for microscopic cell analysis, and hormone therapies.

Era II medicine is what Dossey and others refer to as mind-body medicine, which is gradually being integrated into traditional physical medicine applications. Mind-body medicine asserts that our mind plays an integral role in illness and the recovery from illness and disease. The treatments used in Era II medicine are many and varied, including hypnotherapy, biofeedback, counseling, and various relaxation and imagery techniques. One exciting new field of research is psychoneuroimmunology, which focuses on researching how specific stressors can generate profound health consequences. Many researchers are now suggesting that stress— especially chronic stress—directly affects our immune system in significant and measurable ways, preventing the mind-body system from being able to rebalance itself to achieve and maintain homeostasis. We now know that emotions such as anger, fear, anxiety and prolonged grief cause measurable physiological reactions in our nervous system that can ultimately impair immune function. This is called immunosuppression and can result in otherwise healthy people coming down with pneumonia, generating ulcers or other digestive disorders, contracting cancer and even dying shortly after the death of a long-time spouse (sometimes called the broken heart syndrome).

These treatment approaches have two important characteristics in common. First, they all address imbalances in the mind-body relationship. Second, many of these therapies are now accepted by the traditional medical community—medical doctors often refer their patients to practitioners who use these techniques, and many health insurance plans cover the costs of these treatments.

The proven effectiveness of these mind-body approaches strongly suggests that the mind has causal, or at least influential, powers *within the individual.* Thus, it is now known (and there is growing acceptance) that consciousness is a significant factor in the development of disease and illness as well as in recovery. When doctors tell their patients that their heartburn, insomnia or migraine headaches are psychosomatic or induced by stress, they are acknowledging a fundamental principle of Era II medicine—that what happens in the mind contributes to the

> Consciousness is a significant factor in the development of disease and illness as well as in recovery.

development of disease and illness. Rather than simply prescribing drugs, doctors may refer patients to biofeedback treatment, or recommend that they meditate twice a day. Thus, these doctors are acknowledging that the mind contributes to the patient's recovery.

Era III medicine

According to Dr. Dossey, Western society is now beginning to move toward Era III medicine, in which we acknowledge and accept an entirely new paradigm for healing. Dossey calls Era III medicine *nonlocal* medicine or *eternity* medicine. This framework extends the Era II concept of the mind-body by recognizing that the effects of the mind—consciousness—can cause physical changes *between* individuals as well as within an individual. Dossey states that the

> mind is not completely localized to points in space (brains or bodies) or time (present moment or single lifetimes). Mind is unbounded in space and time and thus is ultimately unitary or one. Healing at a distance is possible . . . [and] not describable by classical concepts of space-time or matter-energy.[1]

Dossey goes on to say that nonlocal medicine

> grants the mind freedom to roam freely in space and time. In Era III, the mind is more than the brain; it can do things brains can't do, such as acting remotely from the body and venturing outside the present.[2]

If the mind is not bound by space and time, it is everywhere always (and thus ultimately One rather than "first here, and then over there"), and all forms of nonlocal intentionality, such as distant healing and prayer, become possible. This suggests that our mind (or at least a part of our consciousness) can affect things outside of our body, even another person who is on the other side of the world.

Have you ever wondered about the unlimited power to influence others described in the stories and myths ascribed to the gods and where these stories originated, psychological theories aside? Many myth stories appear to be fictitious, since they often describe supernatural powers wielded by imaginary beings characterized as gods or goddesses. But there are many accounts of unusual feats of consciousness described in the scriptural literature of many ancient religious traditions, including indigenous-based shamanistic cultures. While these descriptions can be judged to be apocryphal or without any kind of determinable basis of fact, contemporary scientific experimental research is suggesting that many of these supernatural attributes are, in fact, realizable.

At first, this idea of the mind being able to roam freely without regard for time or space may seem more fantasy than reality. But the idea of nonlocal mind is not a new one. Spiritual masters from Jesus to Paramahansa Yogananda have taught that we are both body and spirit, local and nonlocal.

To fully understand the concept of the nonlocal mind, you must get beyond the conventional Western thinking that each of us is separate from other people and contained solely within our physical body. In fact, we are separate physically, but all our consciousness, that ephemeral energy that makes up the fundamental composition of what we call our mind and spirit, is interconnected to form One universal field, a concept not dissimilar to Carl Jung's collective unconscious mind. Also, keep in mind that when we use the power of nonlocal intentionality, we are not really sending our thoughts from "here" to a destination somewhere "way over there," since our concept of physical space is not relevant to the nonlocal mind. A common example is when you are looking at someone from your car and that person turns his head directly at you, as if your focused attention or consciousness just penetrated his awareness and felt intrusive to him. This is a classic example of the nonlocal mind at work.

Dossey has identified three characteristics that are common to nonlocal events:

> They are said to be *unmediated* (the distant changes
> do not depend on the transmission of energy or on
> any sort of energetic signal); they are *unmitigated* (the
> strength of the changes does not become weaker with

increasing distance); and they are *immediate* (the distinct changes take place simultaneously).[3]

Now let's look briefly at the evidence that has been found to support the existence and effectiveness of nonlocal events.

The power of prayer—Compassion in action

Let's begin by looking at the power of prayer, which is perhaps the best example of the nonlocal mind in action. Prayer is familiar to nearly everyone from every culture and religious tradition, because it is an integral part of all religious practice.

There are many varieties of prayer, from singing hymns as a group to privately asking for divine intervention. Some prayers are a way to ask the Divine for help to bring about a very specific outcome for an individual—these are prayers of petition or intercession. A prayer to help someone heal asks for the power and miraculous energy of the Absolute or Divine to help in generating positive and healing outcomes for that person. When we are praying, however we may conceive of it, we are trying to communicate with the Divine from our heart so that the power of love and compassion will bring about positive transformation and healing. Other prayers are more open-ended and nondirected. An example of this type of prayer is "May the best outcome prevail," or "Thy will be done."[4]

All prayers acknowledge our relationship with something invisible, mysterious, influential and more powerful than us. Although the impulse to ask for help from a cosmic benefactor may seem irrational, humans continue to regularly use this ancient practice that reflects a basic and essential part of who we are. In poll after poll, Americans confirm that prayer is a major part of the fabric of their lives, regardless of religion, creed, level of education or family background. Yet, many people are skeptical about the effectiveness of prayer, and believe that asking an invisible

God for things is irrational. Is there a way that science can help us understand whether prayer really works?

The answer is yes. Clinical research on the effects of distant healing has been going on for a number of decades. In December 1997, nearly one hundred researchers from universities throughout the United States gathered at a landmark conference at Harvard to share the results of their studies on nonlocal or distant healing. All their research studies had a singular goal—to determine if individuals could mentally create healing outcomes for people who were unaware they were being targeted for healing at a distance.

> The researchers described this effort in various ways. Some called it "prayer," while others preferred "distant intentionality," "empathic concern," or some other more secular-sounding terminology. All the studies were ventures into Era III medicine and nonlocal mind—the capacity of human consciousness to function outside the confines of the individual brain and body.[5]

Of the many fascinating studies reviewed, I would like to highlight two in particular that stand out as moving examples of how the mind creates healing responses from a distance.

Perhaps the most well known study is that directed by cardiologist Randolph Byrd in 1988. The study was conducted at San Francisco General Hospital over a ten-month period. A computer assigned 393 cardiac surgery patients to participate in the experiment. Of those, 192 were selected to be prayed for after their surgeries; the remaining 201 patients were not prayed for. As is common in well-controlled research studies, Byrd used randomization and double-blind administration so that none of the nurses, doctors and patients who participated knew who was or was not being prayed for. The people who volunteered to pray included many Roman Catholic and Protestant groups from across the country. Each person praying was given the first names of the patients and a short description of their diagnoses and current conditions. They were asked simply to pray each day in whatever way they thought best. "Each person prayed for many different patients," Byrd explained, and "each patient in the experiment had between five and seven people praying for him or her."[6]

The results were remarkable. Patients in the prayed-for group benefited in a number of ways compared to those in the not-prayed-for group. Differences between the two groups included the following:

- On average, patients in the prayed-for group had fewer than half the post-surgical complications than patients who were not prayed for, and their surgical incisions healed faster.
- Prayed-for patients were five times less likely to require antibiotics.
- Prayed-for patients were three times less likely to develop pulmonary edema, a condition in which the lungs fill with fluid because the heart is not pumping properly.
- None of the prayed-for patients needed endotracheal intubation (in which an artificial airway is inserted in the throat and attached to a mechanical ventilator), while twelve in the not-prayed-for group required mechanical ventilatory support.
- Fewer patients in the prayed-for group died.[7]

The second study I want to comment on was presented at the same Harvard conference in 1997. The researcher was Father Sean O'Laoire, a Catholic priest and psychologist. O'Laoire selected 406 people and divided them into two groups—one group was prayed for and the other was not. All 406 participants were pre-tested to measure their responses to questions in eleven categories related to self-esteem, depression and anxiety. O'Laoire also collected data on the ninety people who were responsible for the praying. Again, as in the Byrd study, he used a controlled, double-blind procedure so that no one knew who was and was not being prayed for. After the testing period, O'Laoire measured the participants on the same eleven categories. The subjects who had been prayed for improved in all eleven categories. *But the most interesting result related to those who were doing the praying. They improved even more than those who were prayed for!*[8]

What does all this have to do with caregivers learning to take better care of themselves while attending to others in need? Simply stated, the evidence from these two studies seems to indicate that the thoughts we direct at another person can create positive physiological, mental and emotional changes in that individual. A major theme in these two experiments on the power of prayer is that those who did the praying not only created positive change for their subjects, but they themselves felt better emotionally for their efforts.

> *But the most interesting result related to those who were doing the praying. They improved even more than those who were prayed for!*

While these studies show how the power of prayer influences the caregiver or helper (the person doing the praying) and the person being prayed for, they also tend to corroborate Dossey's thesis about nonlocal medicine.

For a more detailed discussion on how caregivers can use prayer to help themselves and the person they are helping, see Chapter 12.

The power of intention—Applied consciousness

Ongoing scientific research is providing profound evidence for the power of intention. While this has become a very popular subject for new age and popular culture theorists and authors, intention is more than powerfully focused determination to generate a specific result. As I said in my first book,

Consider the possibility that intention is not something
which you create by your will alone but is instead a force
that exists in the universe as an invisible and infinite
field of energy, responsive to your every thought.[9]

The Princeton Engineering Anomalies Research facility
(PEAR) has been investigating this phenomenon for many years.
PEAR was founded by Robert G. Jahn, a former dean of Princeton's
engineering department. The results of the PEAR experiments
support Dossey's assertion that distance does not affect the mind's
power to apply consciousness to influence events that occur outside
the body.

Many of the PEAR experiments have used electronic random-event generators. These generators are programmed so that
their output is completely random—an electronic equivalent of
somebody flipping coins. PEAR has used a variety of experimental
designs, but one they have used often involves a line moving randomly above and below the midpoint on a computer screen. A
movement above the line reflects the random-event generator's
pluses, while a movement below the line reflects the minuses. In
general, because the generator's output is a random combination
of pluses and minuses, the fluctuating line spends equal time
above and below the screen's midpoint.

The person participating in the experiment is asked to try to
mentally push the line to keep it either above or below the line.
In other words, they use the power of their mind to "intend"
that the computer generate more pluses or more minuses. These
studies found that the random-event generator consistently
responded to the thoughts and intentions of the participants.
Moreover, it didn't matter whether the person trying to influence
the generator was directly in front of the computer screen or
somewhere on the other side of the world. "Over the past two
decades the PEAR researchers have observed *millions* of trials in
which individuals try mentally to influence some physical phe-

nomenon at a distance—the largest database on the subject in the history of science."[10]

Does water harbor memory?

Since the late 1980s, a number of researchers have been trying to determine whether water can "imprint" the energetic influences to which it has been exposed. In a controversial article published in 1988 in *Nature*,[11] a French immunologist named Dr. Jacques Benveniste attempted to explain the mechanisms of how homeopathy works. This research paved the way for others to explore this phenomenon.

The more well-known research on the subject of water memory by Japanese researcher Dr. Masaru Emoto has also created quite a stir. In his book *The Hidden Messages in Water*,[12] Dr. Emoto uses special photographic techniques to visually demonstrate how the vibration of our words affects water crystals. Emoto (and other researchers) believe that the universe is constantly vibrating, and that everything generates a unique vibrational frequency. (These assertions are similar to those of quantum physics, which is discussed later in this chapter.) He has developed technology to photograph the crystalline structure of water that has been frozen after being exposed to either positive or negative thoughts or words. He muses on this:

> But how can we interpret the phenomena of crystal formation being affected by words written on paper and shown to water? The written words themselves actually emit a unique vibration that the water is capable of sensing. Water faithfully mirrors all the vibrations created in the world, and changes these vibrations into a form that can be seen with the human eye. When water is shown a written word, it receives it as vibration, and expresses the message in a specific form.[13]

In one experiment, Dr. Emoto wrapped a piece of paper with the words *love* and *gratitude* written on it around a bottle of water. The photographs taken later show that the water crystals formed beautiful hexagonal crystals. In contrast, when he wrapped the same bottle of water with a piece of paper that said *Fool!*, he asserts that the crystals that formed were irregular, ugly and fragmented.[14]

Emoto has also investigated how the power of prayer affects water. He tells the story of a Shinto priest of the Shingon sect who wanted to demonstrate how praying through chanting at the Fujiwara dam in central Japan would purify the water in the lake. Emoto took photographs of the crystals formed from the lake water before the priest chanted. He then videotaped the ritual chanting. When the priest was finished, he and Dr. Emoto chatted. After fifteen minutes, one of the camera crew called to him excitedly.

"This is incredible! The water is getting clearer right in front of our eyes," someone said. And it was absolutely true. You could clearly see that the water was becoming more and more transparent as we looked at it. We were even able to make out the foliage at the bottom of the lake, which had been hidden by the cloudy water.

We next took photographs of crystals. The crystals made with water from before the incantation were distorted, and looked like the face of someone in great pain. But the crystals from the water taken after the incantation were complete and grand. Within one hexagonal shape there was a smaller hexagonal shape, all enclosed by a halo-like pattern of light.[15]

More recently, new research from the Aerospace Institute of the University of Stuttgart and from other researchers is attempting to corroborate the theory that water does indeed have a memory.[16]

The point I want to highlight is the possibility that the priest's prayers changed the structure of the water to the extent that the effects were visible to the naked eye within fifteen minutes and were not simply an anomaly. Water that was dirty and cloudy became blessed water through the efforts of spiritual prayer. If verifiably true, this is another example of how the power of intention and of prayer—the healing power of love—affects our physical reality.

In the summer of 2010, oil was spewing forth from the catastrophic BP Deepwater Horizon well in the gulf of Mexico, eventually polluting the ocean and inland estuaries with over 155 million gallons of crude oil.[17] No doubt there will be more disastrous oil spills if we continue using deep-water drilling. We also know that many ocean trawlers and other commercial ships dump their toxic waste deep in the oceans, polluting our ecosystems. If we all pray or visualize and set our intent for the dissolution of these toxic wastes and the healing of the water, the research results discussed above support the real possibility that we can collectively create a significant shift in the global field that we are all connected to that will result in positive outcomes supporting a clean environment. Expanding on this possibility, why limit our prayers and healing intentions to just the environment?

As I hope you're beginning to appreciate and consider, applied consciousness through the intentional application of our thoughts is continually demonstrating that *we not only **can** transform and change—we **are** creating those transformations, both inside and outside of ourselves.* This has profound implications for the relevance of nonlocal events to caregivers and their clients.

The power of meditation—Self-coherence and group coherence

The third type of nonlocal power that we all have is the power to achieve self- and group coherence by meditating. In this context, we use the term *coherence* to mean harmony or optimal balance.

Research done by Dean I. Radin, Jannine M. Rebman and Maikwe P. Cross is helpful in understanding and appreciating this idea of coherence. Based on some of their research, they concluded that consciousness is not only nonlocal. Consciousness is an "ordering principle"; that is, individuals can increase their level of inner coherence and the level of coherence in the world outside of themselves. "It can insert information into disorganized or random systems and create higher degrees of order."[18] This can be achieved by both individuals and larger collectives or groups.

When an individual is ill or emotionally distraught, one can say that they are out of harmony with themselves or that they lack inner coherence. Thus, they are a kind of disorganized system that would benefit from "higher degrees of order."

Similarly, groups of people, including entire cities and countries, can be disorganized systems. Physicist Dr. John Hagelin, who is now affiliated with Maharishi University, where transcendental meditation (TM) is taught, is interested in whether consciousness affects world peace. He has conducted experiments in which he tested whether the power of a group of people meditating can increase the degree of coherence in a city. Hagelin conducted a study in the summer of 1993 in Washington, DC. Police data show that, in general, crime rates are higher in summer, in large measure because of the extreme heat and the toll it takes on the urban population who are spending more time out-of-doors. Throughout June and July of that summer, Hagelin brought into the city between 2500 and 4000 practicing meditators (some of whom were new to meditation and trained upon arrival), whose job was to meditate regularly during that period of time. Halfway through the experiment, there was a distinct and highly statistically significant drop in crime compared to expected rates based on previous data, weather conditions, and a variety of other factors. They collaborated with the local police department, the FBI, and 24 leading, independent criminologists and social scientists

> Consciousness is an "ordering principle."

from major institutions, including the University of Maryland, the University of Texas and Temple University, who used highly sophisticated research tools to control for variables such as weather. Everyone ended up agreeing on the language, the analysis, and the results, and those results were quite astonishing. They had predicted a 20 percent drop in crime, and achieved a 25 percent drop.[19]

What impressed Hagelin enormously was that by creating group coherence through a consciousness application (meditation) using only a few thousand people, a significant number of people in a city with a population of about one and a half million were positively influenced.

A similar study had been conducted during the height of the Israel-Lebanon war in the 1980s. The results were published in Yale University's *Journal of Conflict Resolution*.[20] In that study, the researchers found that

> on days when the numbers of meditators were largest (and also on the subsequent days), levels of conflict were markedly reduced—by about 80 percent overall. This turned out to be a statistically significant effect and also a surprising one, because there were only about 600 to 800 people meditating in the midst of this entire conflict and the highly stressed surrounding population.[21]

Over the next two and a half years, seven more experiments were done on the effects of group meditation on the Israel-Lebanon conflict. The meditators met in Israel, Lebanon, Europe and other parts of the world. Hagelin reports that

> In each case, when the size of the group reached the threshold that was predicted (based on previous research) to have an effect, there was a marked and statistically significant reduction of violence. We have also found in

other studies that in the geographic vicinity of such a meditating group, people experienced physiological changes—increased EEG coherence, reduced plasma cortisol, increased blood levels of serotonin, biochemical changes, and neurophysiological changes—as if *they* were meditating.[22]

It is important to emphasize that the TM meditators did not focus on the intention to reduce crime or violence in Washington, DC, or the Middle East. Instead, they were simply following their prescribed meditation practice of repeating a mantra in order to create individual coherence within themselves. As a consequence of their collective consciousness extending beyond their individual selves (that is, nonlocally), the "ordering power" of their collective field of coherence "inserted information and order" into the disorganized systems of agitation and conflict. In turn, this created measurable reductions in the amount of chaotic and violent behavior. As well, the physiological indicators of stress were significantly reduced among the people influenced by the group of meditators.

In other words, *as the consciousness of individuals and groups becomes more coherent, it helps to bring about measurable, positive shifts in the surrounding environment.* As Radin, Rebman and Cross have identified, "Coherence among individuals is important in the ordering power of consciousness. Coherence may be expressed as love, empathy, caring, unity, oneness and connectedness."[23]

It is interesting to note that the prayer, intention, and meditation studies summarized above demonstrate that the people being affected by the healing intentions of others do not have to be aware that they are the recipients of these intentions. This suggests that people do not have to be open in any particular way to receive the healing benefits of another's loving intentions.

One of the most important aspects of these findings is that they convincingly challenge the contention that nonlocal healing occurs due to the placebo effect. The placebo effect, which is well documented through medical research, is an improvement to a subject's health that happens because the subject expects it to happen. The placebo effect has been attributed to the power of the subject's positive belief—in other words, the claim is that the placebo effect is self-created. But the studies done on nonlocal healing refute the

> The people being affected by the healing intentions of others do not have to be aware that they are the recipients of these intentions.

idea that the placebo effect is responsible for the results. Some of the more than 130 well-documented double-blind research studies have proven that distant healing works on mice, seeds, bacteria, fungi and yeast cells under controlled laboratory conditions.[24] These results must exclude the placebo effect as an explanation for the results obtained since mice, seeds, and yeast cells cannot think positively or "expect" anything to happen.

The quantum physics perspective

While spiritually based people believe that love is the power and force throughout the cosmos that makes nonlocal events possible, the emerging field of quantum physics uses language such as *particles* and *waves* to explain these events. In this paradigm, these particles and waves have unique vibratory frequencies that communicate to the world, making up all that is. The mystifying wrinkle is that this new science asserts that *we are composed of these particles and waves.* Even when we are just observers of what is happening around us, the unique vibratory or frequency signature of each individual influences the outcomes in their reality. Thus, whether we are consciously intentional with our thoughts or not, we unwittingly reduce the infinite possibilities or future outcomes into a single probability just by paying attention to certain things but not others.

One of the fundamental laws of quantum physics says that an event in the subatomic world exists in all possible states until the act of observing or measuring it "freezes" it, or pins it down, to a single state. This process is technically known as the collapse of the wave function, where the "wave function" means the state of all possibilities.[25]

Clearly, this abstract idea challenges the belief that everything in the universe occurs randomly—rather, our consciousness is the agent of creative transformation. Repeated well-documented experiments in the field of quantum physics have shown that you and I, the living and participating observers, create the shifts in the "quantum field" that allow our consciousness (that is, our thoughts) to turn what began as ideas into concrete manifestation. Quantum physicists call this "the observer effect."

Does the concept of the observer effect mean that the spiritual explanations for nonlocal events are wrong? Not at all—qigong masters have known for many years that "energy flows where attention goes," and there is now a large body of experimental evidence gathered over many years that proves conclusively that nonlocal intention or intercessory prayer has measurable positive outcomes. Yet, many people find the quantum physics explanation about subatomic particles and waves easier to accept because it appears more scientifically based and thus somehow more understandable or legitimate.

Of course, to say that repeated double-blind randomized experiments prove that prayer, intentions and meditation work is not to say that anyone really knows *how* they work. To know that, we would need a viable and understandable explanation of how consciousness works, and for now, that continues to be part of the Great Mystery. The nonlocal event experiments are simply the best way that scientists have been able to eliminate variables that interfere with objectivity and reproducibility.

Implications for high-intensity relaters

As the evidence summarized in this chapter clearly shows, by virtue of our nonlocal nature we affect and are affected by everyone around us (and beyond our immediate sphere). *We are always interconnected with and influencing others, and our thought forms affect others, whether we realize it or not.* That is why it's so important for you to be aware of and mindful of your thoughts and reactions. Through this mindfulness, you will be able to choose how you want to affect the world in general as well as the person you are caring for in particular.

> Our consciousness is the agent of creative transformation.

By taking seriously Dossey's three characteristics of nonlocal events (stated above), you have the power to transform the way you see your role as a helper or caregiver and what is required of you. After all, this new Era III medicine paradigm suggests that you can profoundly affect the healing outcomes of your clients by maintaining an attitude of unconditional love and compassion toward them, praying for them, and visualizing them as being already healed. For example, by clearly visualizing a healing image, such as golden light or a beautiful violet rose superimposed on a person, you can consciously insert higher degrees of order to create greater coherence in that person, whether he's right in front of you or many miles away.

Clearly, as caregivers we can use our nonlocal nature for the benefit of others. But just as importantly, we can use it to help us maintain our own well-being. Intentionally inserting information and order into disorganized systems in order to heal has radical implications for the self-care management of caregivers. When you are actively praying for others or in

> You can profoundly affect the healing outcomes of your clients by maintaining an attitude of unconditional love and compassion toward them.

a prayerful state of mind, by definition you are breaking down the boundaries that separate you from others. As a result, your own feelings of anomie and of being isolated from others are eased. This is a natural result of your deepening empathic concern, internal quiet and serenity, and being in a state of compassion and greater interconnectedness. Thus, by consciously, actively intending to help others heal, your attitude and thoughts support the healing of others and bring you to greater personal wellness and self-care.

> By consciously, actively intending to help others heal, your attitude and thoughts support the healing of others and bring you to greater personal wellness and self-care.

As your understanding of your nonlocal nature grows and you begin to use it consciously in a positive way, you will improve the health of both you and your client. Thus, healing will go beyond your separate selves to become a truly shared experience.

Questions and Exercises

1. Reflect on how "prayerful" you are. Do you pray daily as a spiritual practice, or only when you believe that others need extra help? Do you believe that you must be affiliated with a religious group or congregation in order to feel comfortable praying for another person? Consider praying today for someone who you know really could use the help.

2. Where does your belief in the efficacy of prayer come from? Is it faith-based, having emerged from your religious tradition? Or is it based on your own, consistently validated experience? Perhaps you orient more toward a humanistic or even science-based materialist orientation. Maybe you're even an atheist. Discuss praying with two or three people you know and find out what others believe. Make sure not to fall into a polarizing

and judgmental attitude. Attempt to clarify your own thoughts about whether you believe prayer works.

3. Have you ever experienced turning around to look at someone only to discover that they had been staring at you? Has the opposite experience ever happened to you when you were looking at someone from a distance? Did you look away because you believed they felt you were intruding on them? Experiment on your own to find out if this kind of phenomenon happens to you. If so, consider that your mind may have more influence than you ever thought about before. Consider that parts of your consciousness that are not available to your normal awareness are working and providing information to you all the time you just have to pay more attention to become more aware of them.

4. Have you tried meditating? Do you meditate as part of your daily routine? If you do, is it easy for you, or does it continue to be a challenge? Do your thoughts actually get quieter or more agitated? What do you notice about your mood and self-awareness when you are finished? Do you feel more in harmony with yourself? with others? Do you notice anyone you live or work with responding to you any differently, as if they might mysteriously be in greater harmony with you?

CHAPTER

5

The Awakening Self

Let's briefly review some of our discussions so far as they relate to empathy. In Chapter 2, we defined *empathy* as the ability to know what another person is feeling emotionally and somatically. I also discussed that a major characteristic of people who personify the "helper personality"—which I call the high-intensity relater—is that they are highly empathic. It is my assertion that most high-intensity relaters have keen interpersonal intelligence and sensitivity that allows them to support others with élan and derive great personal satisfaction from their interactions. Thus, high-intensity relaters are better qualified than most to help others.

In this chapter, we look at empathy in greater depth, and begin to discuss measures that high-intensity relaters can and should take to protect themselves from being overwhelmed by their heightened empathic abilities.

Unconscious empathy can be damaging to your health and well-being

The intricacies and mechanics of empathy are complex and seemingly mysterious. Social scientists have said that empathy is essential for our very survival, because empathy makes us aware of the experiences and motives of others. In fact, through empathy we vicariously experience the feelings and thoughts of others. When we are relating to another person and experiencing empathy, we are in a place of deep rapport with that person's experience in the moment.

Empathy can be a very positive experience. We feel drawn to be around people who are upbeat, because some of their ebullient attitude and energy seems to rub off on us. You have probably experienced "catching" a high from another person's buoyant mood—it can be exhilarating. But being empathic means that you can also "catch" negative feeling states and attitudes and feel contaminated by others. Being around a severely depressed person can drain the life force energy right out of you and leave you feeling depleted. Encounters with people who radiate negative thoughts and feelings can be emotionally toxic and generate emotional and physical symptoms in us.

Feelings and moods—both positive and negative—are contagious. Essentially, you are "infected" by the feeling states of the people around you. Empathy can also be a nonlocal phenomenon (see Chapter 4), since you don't have to be physically close to someone to catch their mood. We can even empathize with fictional characters, such as when we have feelings of sadness that match a character's grief on the screen or in a novel.

Of the many dynamics happening between people—especially if at least one of them is a high-intensity relater—empathy stands out as a defining component of the interpersonal experience. In the helping context, empathy works both ways. On the positive side, empathy is what allows caregivers to be so supportive of others. For example, therapists who are deeply empathic have been described as being incredibly intuitive, since they seem to read their clients' thoughts and know exactly what and how they are feeling. But at the same time, the helping relationship is especially challenging because helpers are often working with individuals in dire need who are in a great deal of pain. When high-intensity relaters vic-

> Essentially, you are "infected" by the feeling states of the people around you.

ariously experience their client's pain, depression, and feelings of hopelessness, their acute empathic sensitivity can blindside them and suck them down into a black hole of toxic emotions and deteriorating physical health like an unsuspecting undertow at a seemingly tranquil beach.

I believe that *the* essential component of caregiver self-care is to first become conscious of your empathic process, and then learn how to control it to avoid being overwhelmed by it.

Before you can learn how to bring *your* empathic process into your conscious awareness, you will need to understand empathy in more depth. What is the mechanism by which we catch the feelings of others? How might empathy cause distress for the caregiver or helper? What role does empathy play in the fatigue, illness or burnout that high-intensity relaters are so susceptible to? Why do so many in the helping professions fall ill?

> I believe that *the* essential component of caregiver self-care is to first become conscious of your empathic process, and then learn how to control it to avoid being overwhelmed by it.

Essentially, what goes on in the interpersonal field between the caregiver and the person being helped is subtle to the point of being almost imperceptible. When a caregiver and her client come together, an enormous exchange of information occurs on multiple levels. This happens throughout their time together and there is ongoing mutual influence. This is happening simultaneously at the conscious, unconscious and somatic levels.

Unconscious mimicry and rapport

The exchange of emotional information that is at the foundation of our feelings of empathy is mostly unconscious. We communicate our thoughts and intellectual insights through our words, and thus we are fully conscious that this part of the information exchange is happening. But our emotions and moods are communicated to others very differently, and most people are not consciously aware of the exchange of this information. Our emotions and moods are conveyed by the (primarily) nonverbal language of our body. In fact, modern communication research indicates that over 90 percent of emotional messaging is nonverbal.[1] Understanding the power of this nonverbal transmission of emotions and recognizing it in the moment are crucial self-care skills for caregivers to develop.

Many high-intensity relaters are so attuned to the feelings of others that they actually *physically experience* the moods of others.

> Many high-intensity relaters are so attuned to the feelings of others that they actually *physically experience* the moods of others.

How does this happen? The answer is that we unconsciously imitate or mimic all varieties of physical and postural movements in our interactions with others. Researchers have determined that facial mimicry often occurs out of our awareness, as if by reflex. They speculate that this phenomenon is an evolutionary development that is an important aspect of the social glue that helps to maintain group cohesion. It has also been suggested that, in our everyday encounters with others, we tend to unconsciously and continuously move in synch with the facial expressions, vocal tones, movements, postures and even emotional tones of others.

When you unconsciously mimic another person's posture, facial expression and/or physical movements, new information is routed to your brain and autonomic nervous system. This information actually generates within you the emotions that the other person's body is unconsciously conveying. This is due to the physiological changes that happen instantaneously throughout your body, such as changes to your heart rate and fluctuations in your skin temperature.[2] For example, when another person's body language and tone of voice indicate that they feel depressed and hopeless, you unconsciously begin to mimic that body language and tone. These changes in your movements and tone then trigger changes in your brain and autonomic nervous system that start to make *you* feel depressed and hopeless. This process, in essence, is what we call empathy.

In our society, we usually consider empathy to be a positive trait in people. Those who empathize with others are seen as thoughtful, caring and compassionate. But the difficulty is that because this physical process of feeling empathy occurs largely outside our conscious awareness, it's very difficult to turn off your empathy.

Emotional contagion

Social scientist Elaine Hatfield and her colleagues use the term *emotional contagion* for a concept that is very similar to empathy. According to them, the emotions and moods that we feel are often similar to and influenced by the emotions and moods of other people.[3] Hatfield found that emotional contagion occurs not just within Western European societies but cross-culturally. Thus, emotional contagion, wherein we lose our personal emotional autonomy and become swept up in the emotional experience of others, is an inherently human experience—it can happen to anyone.

Unconscious empathy causes emotional contagion. For helpers and caregivers, this is the down side of empathy, and its consequences are profoundly experienced on a somatic level. Since all emotions are contagious—those that we would describe as pleasant as well as those that are not—just what is at work here? *It is a synchrony that is always happening as one person's body is empathizing with another's.* Mimicking another person's posture, vocalizations or movements usually results in empathizing with that person's physical and emotional state of being. This happens primarily through facial and postural mirroring, so it is called *somatic empathy.* "Each feeling (happy, sad, angry, surprised, afraid, etc.) has a specific, observable somatic manifestation ... numerous studies confirm that people unconsciously mirror each other all the time."[4]

For a moment, let's compare emotional contagion with what happens when a person is hypnotized. A person under hypnosis does and says things that normally they would not, and this process is unconscious—when he "wakes up," he is frequently unaware of what he said and did while under hypnosis. Emotional contagion is also unconscious—you are influenced by other people's feelings and moods even though you are not aware of it happening. In both hypnosis and emotional contagion, emotional states are often being induced in the person without his or her conscious awareness. This induction elicits the same feelings that the other person is experiencing.

Interestingly, and perhaps more perniciously, a caregiver's or helper's unconscious empathy also elicits the associated autonomic nervous system reactions that the other person is experiencing. This means that when emotional contagion is occurring, the high-intensity relater experiences a transfer of the body sensations and feelings that the person being helped is experiencing in that moment. If the client is experiencing fear, panic or trauma, the caregiver "catches" those feelings from the client and experiences them at the level of autonomic nervous system changes.

> If the client is experiencing fear, panic or trauma, the caregiver "catches" those feelings from the client and experiences them at the level of autonomic nervous system changes.

Carol (Part 1)

Carol is a clinical psychologist who, when I met her, had been working at a well-regarded mental health clinic for 15 years. The psychologists who worked there treated a diverse population of clients, and Carol worked with families, teenagers, and individual adults of both genders.

Carol's supervisor had been exposed to some of the energy-based therapies and techniques that I teach and use. About three years ago, the supervisor suggested that Carol come to me for some specialized training in how to help her clients who had post-traumatic stress disorder (PTSD). During our third session, Carol disclosed to me that she was having particular difficulties treating one client, Sarah. Carol had been working with Sarah for six months, and Carol had recently begun to suspect that their sessions together were generating all kinds of somatic problems for Carol. In addition, Carol had begun to experience persistent anxiety that carried over into the rest of her life, and she believed that this anxiety was somehow related to her working with Sarah.

Sarah, who was in her mid-thirties, had been diagnosed with adult onset multiple sclerosis (MS) two years before. She had always been a runner and a fitness buff, but she could no longer run on a daily basis. In fact, she had numbness in her extremities and at times a lack of coordination even while walking. Essentially, Sarah was experiencing a progressive loss of normal function, and she was continuously grieving this enormous loss. During her sessions with Carol, Sarah often broke down and cried uncontrollably for up to five minutes at a time.

As Carol and I talked, she told me that she was okay sitting with Sarah in a supportive manner as Sarah was crying. But one day, after Carol had been treating Sarah for about two months, Carol noticed that she was experiencing increasing anxiety and a tingling sensation in her left leg after some of her sessions with Sarah, and these symptoms would persist for hours (and, more recently, for days) at a time. Her arms and legs often felt cold after Sarah described how upsetting it was to have difficulty just walking normally, whereas before she regularly ran for up to forty minutes at a time.

Although Carol wasn't absolutely certain that Sarah was the cause of her symptoms, she became suspicious when the anxiety and tingling seemed to recur after sessions with Sarah. Carol went to her family physician, who found that there was nothing wrong physically. The best the physician could do for Carol was prescribe anti-anxiety medication.

As I got to know her better, Carol admitted that one of the reasons she believed she was such an effective clinical psychologist was because she was "deeply empathetic" with her clients. Even as a child, she "just knew" what other people were feeling. She described her ability as being a second sense or "constant emotional tracking radar" that was unerringly accurate. This ability was the main reason for Carol choosing psychology as a college major and eventually as a career. Carol is a classic high-intensity relater.

As Sarah was communicating so emotionally her grief and sadness about her loss of function, Carol *unconsciously* felt into Sarah's physical experience as a way to more deeply know and understand Sarah's physical suffering. Without realizing it, Carol was vicariously experiencing Sarah's numbness and taking that knowing right into her own physical body and nervous system. Carol's tingling, which was becoming increasingly distracting and worrisome, was *information* being encoded somatically about Sarah's physical experience of MS. In her deeply compassionate attempt to understand Sarah's experience, Carol was essentially absorbing Sarah's MS symptoms. Since she was doing so *unconsciously*, Carol was becoming increasingly alarmed about her own health.

The interplay between Carol and Sarah is an excellent example of emotional contagion. Later in this chapter, I explain what strategies Carol used to recover from this contagion and sufficiently protect herself while she continued working with Sara

The unconscious empathic identification with another person is a remarkable energetic merging that reflects how we are all integrally and deeply connected with one another. If this ability to transfer and catch moods is inherent or innate in all humans (albeit unconscious), it explains a great deal about what is occurring all the time between and among people in all kinds of social contexts. We are all affected by the empathic process, but high-intensity relaters feel the effects of it more intensely than others. Unfortunately, this poses a significant problem for many caregivers.

> We are all affected by the empathic process, but high-intensity relaters feel the effects of it more intensely than others.

Become conscious of your empathic process

Helpers and caregivers in nearly any role find themselves swimming in the sea of human emotions. For these high-intensity relaters, learning how to consciously manage their empathy is essential for two reasons.

First, bringing your empathic process into your conscious awareness makes you a more effective caregiver. The ability to know another's feelings and apply this "interpersonal intelligence" consciously leads to compassion that allows you to be fully present with the other—it supports your ability to respond to the other, especially when the other is experiencing pain. Conscious empathy supported by self-awareness provides what psychiatrist Daniel Stern calls *interpersonal attunement.*[5] Stern studied mothers interacting with their infants, and discovered that when a mother fully acknowledges and reciprocates an infant's emotions, a wonderful interpersonal dance between infant and mother occurs. This attunement dance has an organic rhythm that enfolds both participants as effortlessly as the ocean waves crashing one after another onto a tropical beach. *For the high-intensity relater, conscious empathy is the most powerful tool you have to provide understanding and support to those in need.*

For caregivers, becoming aware of your empathic process is also essential to ensure your emotional and physical survival. The person you

> *For the high-intensity relater, conscious empathy is the most powerful tool you have to provide understanding and support to those in need.*

are helping is likely experiencing many negative emotions. Through the unconscious processes of mimicry and emotional contagion, it's very likely that you will start generating distressing and uncomfortable physical symptoms, if indeed that is not already happening. When you become conscious of your empathic process, you can prevent the energetic, mental/emotional and somatic problems that may accrue from becoming overidentified with others' moods and emotions.

> Becoming aware of your empathic process is also essential to ensure your emotional and physical survival.

Protect yourself from empathic overidentification with others

Develop second attention awareness

In order to truly be helpful, it is essential that you maintain your relational autonomy, all the while sustaining your sense of staying connected to yourself (and your sense of being in your own power) so that your individual integrity is never compromised. Because of the physical and emotional stress that is present in the relational field when caregivers are supporting others, learning to cultivate what I call a second attention awareness can keep you from losing yourself and being overwhelmed by the other person's emotions.[6]

> Learning to cultivate what I call a second attention awareness can keep you from losing yourself and being overwhelmed by the other person's emotions.

As you learn to pay greater attention to your own experience in the process of relating to and supporting the other, you will develop the ability to separate your feelings from your client's. This will allow you to identify your most vulnerable buttons that certain types of clients push over and over again. Then, you will be able to track the somatic cues that your autonomic nervous system generates. It's the autonomic nervous system that is responsible for the physical reactions that put us into the fight, flight or freeze mode under conditions of stress and when we're feeling threatened.

Cultivating second attention awareness requires ongoing, conscious, multilevel self-monitoring. Instead of becoming overly fixated on your client's needs or narrative (that is, your external reality at the time), the type of dual awareness that I'm talking about requires paying exquisite attention to any signs that your autonomic nervous system is becoming aroused in ways that can be cumulatively debilitating. Signs to look for include

- muscles tensing
- heartbeat becoming more rapid
- extremities becoming cold
- negative or critical thoughts or images starting to intrude in your consciousness
- the feeling of being spaced out, often a clue that you're beginning to dissociate or leave your body.

When you notice that any of these responses are beginning to take you over, it's important to acknowledge that your unconscious empathy is likely creating a dangerous interpersonal trance. No matter how riveting your client's story is or how intensely their expression of their pain might be, you must take immediate action to "unmirror" yourself and break rapport in order to step out of the interpersonal trance that has swept you up and caught you like a powerful river current.

Here are some practical suggestions for how to *consciously* take care of yourself by unmirroring from your client's movements and posture:

1. Keep a glass of water nearby so you can frequently move your eyes away from your client to take a drink.
2. If necessary, excuse yourself to go into another room (such as taking a bathroom break) for a couple of minutes as a way to break contact completely.

3. Consciously changing your breathing is very helpful, particularly as you look away and take a couple of deep breaths.
4. To break your body away from mimicking the posture and movements of your client, deliberately change your body position and move your arms regularly.

Take a mini break to write some notes and collect yourself during the session. Writing notes averts your eyes from your client and breaks the interpersonal trance.

While it may seem rude to break eye contact and compromise your rapport with the person you are helping, doing so enables you to stay the course and support your client. It also affirms to yourself that you are in charge of yourself, even as you stay connected to your client.

Carol (Part 2)

As I helped Carol to reflect on how her helping relationship with Sarah was affecting her, I suspected she might talk about negative or critical thoughts that intruded into her consciousness during and after her sessions with Sarah. She didn't. However, she did describe how images of dried and shrunken cornstalks would suddenly come into her mind after a session with Sarah. Another poignant image that Carol became aware of only when she was with Sarah was from a Vietnam war movie she had seen years before. The image was of soldiers moving through muddy rice paddies under the glaring sun. This image evoked feelings of despair and hopelessness in Carol. She had only noticed these images twice, but they were so vivid that they stuck with her, and they evidently continued to affect her long after these intrusive and distressing images came into her mind. Until we began to work together, Carol did not make the connection that her unconscious empathy or emotional contagion had given rise to the images she saw, the feelings they evoked in her, and the tingling she felt in her legs.

I taught Carol about second attention awareness so she could start paying attention to her mental, emotional and somatic experiences when she was meeting with Sarah. As our sessions progressed, Carol came to recognize that she needed to occasionally break rapport with Sarah by excusing herself to step out of the session for a moment, and by frequently looking away from Sarah to internally reorient to herself and write down some notes. As Carol began taking more and more control over her experience, her anxiety lessened over a period of a few weeks, and the tingling sensations she was experiencing in her leg (mimicking the numbness of Sarah's MS) began to disappear.

Carol later told me that she had come to realize that she needed to work on developing second attention awareness when working with all of her clients so she could feel confident that her health was not being compromised. She also acknowledged that although previously she had believed that it was important to keep eye contact with her clients so they would know she cared about them, she now recognized that she needed to take care of herself first by regularly disengaging eye contact.

Strengthening your inner observer as you cultivate increasingly sensitive second attention awareness takes some time. A good place to start is paying attention to what has been a particularly difficult or persistent stress symptom that tends to emerge in you over the course of the day with clients. Intend from your very first contact of the day to track the progress of this symptom carefully so that eventually you can correlate a particular stimulus from your client with a somatic response in your body. Then, make it a habit to use a variety of the strategies outlined above to temporarily break your empathic connection and bring yourself back to a place of self-awareness and inner calmness.

Over time, you will become increasingly sensitive to what previously were deleterious consequences of unconscious empathy and learn how to prevent them from ever taking hold. Anyone can achieve second attention awareness—it just takes practice. The fact that you are a high-intensity relater makes it especially important for you to develop this skill. Your ability to maintain your health and overall well-being depends on it.

Stay connected to your heart field

Another way to make sure your unconscious empathy doesn't overwhelm you has been suggested by author Penney Peirce. Peirce describes a concept that she calls our "home frequency." She says that when you choose to orient to the frequency of your soul, you begin to stabilize at your home frequency.

> I call it home frequency because it conveys an experience of Home that's as close to heaven on earth as you can get. Your home frequency acts as a compass—when you attune your fluctuating daily *personal vibration* to this most essential, naturally high-frequency energy, your life stabilizes and unfolds with luck, meaning, and enjoyment. . . . Focus on qualities of soul, like cheerfulness, sincerity, innocence, or playful creativity . . . [that have] existed since you were a radiant baby. Think of the you that you love, the way you feel when you're being loving, happy, and generous.[7]

Peirce believes that our home frequency is an energetic reference point we need to consciously refamiliarize ourselves with often, so that when we are thrown off balance by the challenges of daily life and hurtful people, we can take a deep breath, open our heart and return to that place of our essence. This is a subjective experience we can shift into by moving out of our head and into our heart. We need to cultivate this practice consciously, intentionally and on a daily basis.

The power of our physical heart has been scientifically proven to be electromagnetically stronger than the power of the brain. "It is sixty times greater in amplitude than that of the brain, permeates every cell, and can be detected several feet away from the body."[8]

Researchers Rollin McCraty, Raymond Trevor Bradley and Dana Tomasino have determined that "sustained positive emotions appear to give rise to a distinct mode of functioning, which we call 'psychophysiological coherence.'" They elaborate by saying that when in this mode of being, a person experiences "increased efficiency and harmony in the activity and interactions of the body's systems," and a "reduction in internal mental dialogue, reduced perceptions of stress, increased emotional balance, and enhanced mental clarity, intuitive discernment, and cognitive performance."[9] Their research is about our body's "heart field" and what happens to us on multiple levels when we consciously choose to focus on our heart rather than our head when considering our motives for taking action. Once we can consistently recognize and orient to our heart field, we are more prone to stay connected to our home frequency.

It is important to note that since your heart's electromagnetic field emanates significantly beyond your physical body, it can be a positive influence on the people you are helping. When you can sustain this internal first reference point, *being present with another from an attitude of loving kindness becomes more important than anything else you may choose to do.* Clearly, staying connected to your heart field is a fundamental self-care strategy that also directly influences the health and well-being of anyone you are with. The benefits of staying connected to your heart field start with you and expand outward. This is the power of presence, when simply being becomes a blessing to the other as loving presence brings harmony through coherence to those who are out of harmony.

> Staying connected to your heart field is a fundamental self-care strategy that also directly influences the health and well-being of anyone you are with.

(For more on becoming a blessing, see Chapter 12.) A sweet and poignant saying from *The Tao Teh Ching* is helpful in defining the point:

There is no need to run outside
For better seeing,
Nor to peer from a window. Rather abide
At the center of your being;
For the more you leave it, the less you learn.
Search your heart and see
If he is wise who takes each turn:
The way to do is to be.[10]

In practical terms, how can you stay connected to your heart field? When I was training to become a practitioner of neurolinguistic programming (NLP), I learned a technique that can help.

1. Find a memory of a time in your life when you were at your home frequency. Was there a time when you felt connected to your home frequency much of the time (such as being in love for the first time)? Do you have a memory of playing until your feet hurt as a child? Or of the elation you felt as you hiked a beautiful forest trail?

2. Once you have zeroed in on the memory, bring together as many of your senses as you can recall. Pay particular attention to how you felt emotionally at that time, but try also to recall what you heard, saw, smelled and touched.

3. When your memory of that experience is at its most intense, bring together the tip of your ring finger and the tip of your thumb of the same hand. Keep them touching for about thirty seconds, or until the feelings of the positive memory start to dissipate. At that point, disengage your two fingers.

This is called establishing an anchor of the most positive feeling of the memory at your very fingertips. As you practice touching those same two fingertips while reflecting on the feeling of the memory, you are building up and reinforcing a positive association between that simple act and your home frequency. Eventually, you will only have to touch the tips of those fingers together and you will immediately be reconnected to the wonderful, powerful feelings of being at your home frequency. The more frequently you fire off your anchor like this, the more frequently you will be connected to what Peirce calls your home frequency.

Use your second attention awareness to handle "mixed messages"

A particular challenge for high-intensity relaters is being in a situation in which they receive mixed messages from the person they are caring for. When the tone of voice of the sender of information (in this context, the person receiving the care) belies the words they speak, the receiver of the communication gets what is called a double signal.

For example, I was working with a client named James. At the beginning of one of our therapy sessions, I told him that I had allocated ninety minutes, but that we would check in after one hour to see how he was feeling about stopping or continuing. James had a lot of physical pain and anger from a car accident he had been in recently that wasn't his fault. When fifty-five minutes had elapsed, I asked James if he had the energy and desire to continue for another thirty minutes. I received a double signal from him. He said, "Okay, let's continue, even though I'm getting a migraine headache. I have been getting migraines almost continuously since I was smashed into."

What stood out most about James' response was his tone of voice. His voice had gone so soft that I had to strain my ears to hear him. His tone conveyed to me that he felt defeated and exasperated, and it contained within it feelings of desperation, fatigue and pain. He was sending me two separate messages that made me feel conflicted and skeptical. I knew he was angry and in pain from being the victim of a careless driver, and that he wanted to move through his post-traumatic stress because of the depression he had been feeling and the flashbacks that were continually assaulting him. And yet, I was uncertain about whether his true intent really was to continue with our session because of the conflicting feelings conveyed by his mixed message. His tone of voice, which affected me more strongly than his words, led me to suspect that he had reached his threshold and it would be best to stop for the day. Yet his words had told me otherwise.

Double signals such as these are usually conveyed unintentionally, but they are quite common. If you pay attention to your interactions with friends and family, you may notice that the emotional tone in the voice (which is often unconscious) doesn't "match" the conscious part of the message they are intending with their words. The same may be true with respect to someone's hand and body movements versus their words.

Being able to detect mixed messages is an important skill for caregivers to develop. Your client's tone of voice or body movements may indicate an unwillingness to agree to your suggestions, even though their words say yes. Your decision on whether to stay in rapport and mimic their facial expressions and body movements will determine the degree of harmony that you maintain with them during that particular encounter.

> Being able to detect mixed messages is an important skill for caregivers to develop.

Nancy and Matthew

Consider a particular encounter between Nancy, a physical therapist, and Matthew, her client. Matthew has mobility problems as a result of being in a skiing accident a few weeks ago. Nancy suggests to Matthew that he take a walk every day despite the pain in his hip. Matthew responds "Sure, I'll do that," but he has a resentful look on his face.

Matthew has just sent Nancy a mixed message. When this kind of double signaling occurs, it is likely that the person sending the mixed message feels threatened, and is unconsciously sending that dual message as a way to pull away from the other person. In this case, Matthew is probably not aware of his own facial expression. On a conscious level, he is committed to doing everything he can to recover from the accident. On an unconscious level, however, he may dread the thought of walking every day because he believes it will be painful, or he may resent the whole idea of a physical therapist telling him what to do. Unconsciously, he's using his resentful facial expression to put some emotional distance between himself and Nancy.

Meanwhile, Nancy—who is a high-intensity relater—immediately senses that something is wrong. Thanks to her gift of strong emotional empathy, she intuitively picks up Matthew's unconscious ambivalence about going for a daily walk. The mixed message that Matthew has communicated to Nancy creates some tension and confusion in their relationship. Nancy now feels uneasy and uncertain about how to interpret Matthew's real feelings about going for a walk every day.

Nancy has a decision to make. She can choose to stay emotionally attuned from a place of conscious empathy. Or, she can press Matthew about the issue ("Matthew, your voice says yes but your face says no. What's going on?") and risk triggering an open conflict with him.

Ideally, for the sake of herself and her client, Nancy will remind herself to consciously follow her second attention, which will allow her to continue interacting with Matthew in an emotionally attuned, empathic way and thus maintain rapport. To do that, she can ask herself these questions:

1. Has this short exchange with Matthew made me feel physically uncomfortable in any way? For example, is my stomach tensing up? Do I have trouble swallowing? Have my hands gone cold or clammy? If the answer to any of these questions is yes, then my second attention awareness tells me that my body is unconsciously reacting to the conflicting information Matthew is sending me. My body has processed the disconnect between his

words and his facial expression by reacting physically to the mixed message.

2. Do I understand what has just happened in this short exchange? Am I clear on whether Matthew will go on walks as I suggested? If the answer to these questions is no, then my second attention awareness tells me that I am confused by the conflicting information Matthew is sending me. My brain is having difficulty reconciling the messages sent by his words and his facial expression.

If Nancy's attempt to maintain rapport with Matthew is creating unpleasant physical symptoms in her, or if she cannot figure out what Matthew's true intention about walking is, she needs to break that rapport temporarily in order to reconnect with her heart field. She must "step back" momentarily to separate her own experience from Matthew's in order to regain her equilibrium. She could break eye contact with him, busy herself with her notes for a moment, or even excuse herself and leave the room for a minute or two.

Once Nancy is reconnected to her home frequency, she will be able to reorient herself to Matthew. In other words, she will be able to empathize with Matthew's true feelings of fear and resentment. She can then decide if she wants to go slow with him and just leave him alone for now, or bring the issue of his conflicted feelings into the open by attempting to clarify what he really means. By reconnecting with her heart field, Nancy can now continue her session with Matthew from a place of greater understanding.

The interpersonal dance that Daniel Stern describes between infant and mother is also an apt metaphor for the relationship between high-intensity relaters and the people they help. This interpersonal attunement happens when you are sufficiently awake to the myriad dynamics occurring between you and the person you are helping. If you allow yourself to become entranced by the story of the suffering and difficulties of your client, you risk falling into the quicksand of emotional contagion and absorbing their pain, much like what Carol experienced with Sarah. Carol's unconscious empathy allowed her to be consumed by Sarah's total experience of MS, and Carol became a passive participant in the interpersonal dance. She was being led, but did not realize it.

Once Carol awakened to what was going on below the level of her conscious awareness, she began to cultivate second attention awareness. She discovered that she needed to lead in the dance, and so became more active in determining the course of her self-care even as her empathic process stayed current with Sarah. Carol did not diminish or compromise her empathic identification with Sarah. Rather, Carol used the information she obtained through her greater conscious awareness to make better decisions in order to preserve her health and ultimately enjoy the dance of staying interpersonally attuned to Sarah. In this way, Carol became even more supportive of Sarah by staying more present to herself, thus enabling her to stay the course with Sarah for as long as Sarah needed her assistance.

This chapter has outlined the possible pitfalls that are always present when your empathy remains unconscious. With greater understanding and the tools offered here, I am confident you will become even more effective in helping others and, at the same time, take better care of yourself.

Questions and Exercises

1. Try an experiment. The next time you are with a friend or partner, make a conscious effort to mimic that person's facial expressions. In other words, try to mirror back to them the facial expressions they are making. Pay attention to the feeling in the relationship. Does a feeling of greater harmony emerge? If not, keep experimenting and really concentrate on your feelings during these everyday encounters.

2. This time, either with the same person or someone new, copy and reproduce their movements and postures as closely as you can. Try not to be overly obvious. Do you feel yourselves becoming synched up as if you are partners in a wonderful and fascinating interpersonal dance? Do you feel any greater empathy with how the other person is feeling?

3. Try a third experiment. Bring your attention to the mutual field of influence that is always present when two or more people are interacting. Try doing this when you are with someone who is upbeat and sunny. Then, try it with someone who is depressed, sad or negative. How is your feeling state affected or determined by the feelings of the other? Is there any evidence of emotional contagion? If your own energy is affected quickly, this may indicate that you have porous energetic boundaries (see Chapter 7). Stay present with yourself to determine whether your empathy is primarily conscious or unconscious. This awareness will help you to stay healthy and strong when assisting others.

4. Do you have an emotional blind spot? A blind spot makes you vulnerable and creates leaks of your vital energy. Emotional blind spots can be specific to a particular emotion. For example, a blind spot related to grief makes it difficult for you to deal with grief and integrate it healthily. You are more prone to being blindsided by an unexpected or overwhelming response of grief and to being destabilized by it. As you become more aware of your particular emotional vulnerability, your blind spot will be replaced with increased awareness of how to consciously work with each person who embodies and expresses that challenging emotion. With time, your increasing awareness will dissipate this emotional blind spot.

5. The next time you are in conversation with a friend or partner, pay attention to which perceptual channels you notice the

most. During this friendly conversation, are you more sensitive to body sensations, visual images, auditory images and perceptions, feeling states or thoughts? Are you more of a feeler or a thinker? Do you translate the conversation more into images or sounds? Is it easier for you to understand and relate to another person through imagery or through the way things sound? Do you feel more comfortable standing closer or farther away from the other person? Spend some time monitoring how you communicate in a casual and safe interpersonal context. Once you realize what your propensities are, you will have more information available to help you recognize when you start feeling overwhelmed in an emotionally charged interpersonal context, especially when helping others.

6. What are some of the ways that most effectively put you into the state of psychophysiological coherence? For some people it is playing music. For others, it may be meditating, dancing, running or preparing a meal. Think about what activity produces a natural high for you and aligns you with your home frequency. Make some time and do it right now. Make a promise to yourself to do it often!

CHAPTER

6

Prevent Self-Sabotage

You become what you think

Most of us have pervasive thinking patterns that originated in the past (often in early childhood) and that are now so much a part of us that we aren't consciously aware of them. These underlying habits of thinking have a profound effect on our daily thoughts and behavior. What you may not realize is that they also have a profound effect on our physical body. This is because every thought that you think produces a biochemical response in the brain.

> The thoughts that produced the chemicals in the brain allow your body to *feel* exactly the way you were just *thinking*. So every thought produces a chemical that is matched by a feeling in your body.[1]

In other words, *you are physically changed by the very thoughts you generate.* Your thoughts affect your health, your general outlook, and the behavioral choices you make.

> *You are physically changed by the very thoughts you generate.*

Negative thinking patterns frequently result in a physiological pattern of deeply embedded stress chemicals (neuropeptides) that our mind and body have become so familiar with that it's as if we have become addicted to the resultant state of being. While this dysregulation of various stress chemicals is widely recognized in people who have PTSD, it also happens in many other people who are prone to patterns of habitual negative thinking. Similarly, when you are anticipating experiences that bring you pleasure or excitement, neurotransmitters that increase serotonin and dopamine levels in the bloodstream cause positive chemical reactions in the brain.[2]

> Without your conscious awareness, you may be blocking yourself from doing what you really want to do and being who you really want to be.

Pervasive negative thoughts can be the source of self-sabotage that you are not fully aware of consciously. Without your conscious awareness, you may be blocking yourself from doing what you really want to do and being who you really want to be. Your negative thoughts may be preventing you from making positive changes in your life, and they may be compromising your health. The good news is that

the brain doesn't discriminate among thoughts on the neurological level. It takes no more effort to form a positive thought than it does a negative one. Attitudes are simply accumulations of related neural nets, and positive attitudes are as easy to construct as negative ones.[3]

With the many challenges facing caregivers and helpers, maintaining awareness of your thinking habits is essential to prevent the self-sabotage that can push high-intensity relaters into burnout and compassion fatigue.

The three main elements of self-sabotage, which are discussed below, are the influence of your inner critic, your self-limiting beliefs, and the phenomenon of psychoenergetic reversal. Because these can be so damaging to you, a fundamental element of self-care is learning how to recognize them and neutralize them.

Establish an inner observer

The first step in recognizing your self-sabotage is to become aware of and gain control over your own thought patterns by establishing an inner observer that you have an ongoing relationship with. This observer, also known as the meta-communicator (since it is beyond or outside of your normal thinking self), becomes your internal, more objective point of reference. The observer's role is to regularly monitor the negative, critical or doubting inner voice. Your inner observer will also help you monitor and successfully deal with the negative voices that come from outside of you—from other people in your life.

Once your inner observer is firmly in place and you're in proper relationship to it, you will have sufficient expanded awareness to recognize immediately the process that is trying to stop you from succeeding. Your observer is the early warning system that alerts you to intrusive negative and critical influences (whether they are coming from within you or from someone else) that are the basis of your inability to make positive changes in your life. By maintaining your ongoing relationship with your inner observer, you will gradually become able to prevent these mechanisms of self-sabotage from dominating your experience. In the text that follows, I discuss these mechanisms in more detail, and provide you with practical strategies for how to weaken their power over you. As a caregiver or helper who must stay healthy day after day supporting others, it is absolutely essential that you don't get in your own way. Awareness of self-sabotage patterns and having the tools to prevent and dissolve them promotes your ongoing health and well-being. This awareness also supports the emotional energy you need to maintain a positive mental attitude regardless of how challenging your clients are.

The inner critic and self-limiting beliefs

Benjamin Franklin is frequently quoted for his wise observations about human nature. One of his many well-known quotes is about criticism. "Critics are our friends, they tell us our faults." While it is true that critics highlight our faults, I disagree with Mr. Franklin's assessment that critics are who we need to help us in our life. People generally are well aware of their shortcomings and deal with them in different ways. I believe that being constantly barraged by criticism, either coming from outside or inside of ourselves, is ultimately destructive. With all due respect to Mr. Franklin, the quotation above simply misses the point.

Most of us have a critical, doubting part of our thinking process that frequently throws up reasons for why something we are doing won't work. In truth, most of us have a tyrannizing inner critic that intrudes on and interferes with our best intentions for change and self-care. Your inner critic is the little voice that devalues you—it is *not* an objective, judicious voice coming from your left brain's critical thinking process. Your inner critic (which is frequently understood as the internalized voice of a negative inner parent) is a judgmental and negative inner critique that creates your feelings of uncertainty in an effort to avoid change and maintain the status quo. This insidious voice, which can be quite subtle, is relentless in telling you that you won't succeed, you're fooling yourself, or you have failed at something. This constant barrage of discouraging, devaluing thoughts triggers your brain to produce the neuropeptides discussed above, leaving you feeling incompetent and defeated.

In addition, you may have deeply embedded limiting beliefs that are stopping you from making positive changes in your life. For example, deep down, many people have disorientation fears related to creating a new self-identity. These fears may manifest as thoughts such as "This is just who I am and I will never be different." You may also still have the subconscious belief that you are undeserving, for all kinds of untrue reasons. This belief can often be traced back to experiences with negative teachers and shaming parents. Imperatives from family and early religious conditioning may insist that considering your personal goals for your own well-being is selfish and therefore either unethical or unacceptable and damning.

Limiting inner influences such as these are one of the primary reasons that people stay stuck in their current life situation. Their "inner voices" continually remind people of who they are and who they are not. If you always think of yourself as being fat and believe that your weight precludes your involvement in a meaningful personal relationship, I can assure you that you will create this limitation in your life and end up alone.

Sam

Sam, who has been a mental health counselor for almost twenty-four years, has two primary limiting beliefs that his inner critic reminds him of constantly.

The first belief comes from his family's religious background. Altruism and service were the cornerstones of his family's religion, which emphasized helping others in any way possible. Sam internalized the belief that "Other people's needs always come before my own," so he never turns away anyone who seeks counseling. He honors the inner imperative to be of service to as many people as possible by working unusually long hours at the community mental health clinic. In addition to his forty-plus hours at the clinic every week, Sam has a private practice in which he sees clients in the evenings and for much of the day on Saturday. He is an excellent practitioner.

However, now that Sam is nearing sixty-four years old, he has developed adult onset diabetes. He doesn't take the time to eat healthily—he just grabs fast food on the run because it is convenient and he likes the way it satiates him. Additionally, he is exhausted all the time. Sam's doctor has told him that his adrenal glands are depleted, and that he is at risk for chronic fatigue and burnout unless he starts to wind down and consciously exercise more judicious self-care.

Sam is finding it difficult to modify his schedule, even though he admits that he has workaholic tendencies. All of this is because his deeply embedded beliefs to serve others drive him to overwork, to his own detriment. As a high-intensity relater, Sam needs time to withdraw so he can focus on self-care to restore his stores of vital energy, which he is constantly expending with clients. But Sam just doesn't think that his own needs are important.

Sam's other primary self-sabotaging belief arose out of his growing up in a very poor family. His father worked on and off as a construction worker, while his mother stayed at home to take care of Sam and his four siblings. Sam's family was often on public assistance and food stamps, and they received food boxes from their church regularly. Sam heard from his parents that they "never had enough money," and his own perceptions and experiences while growing up reinforced this belief. As Sam worked his way through college and then graduate school, his parents' voices reverberated inside him, constantly reminding him that no matter how hard he seemed to persevere, he just "never had enough money."

Sam did have to endure hardships growing up in a disadvantaged family, but as an adult he could have chosen to challenge these self-limiting beliefs. Instead, his compulsive drive to earn more and more money overcame his occasional awareness that he actually had plenty of money saved and more than enough to live a comfortable life. The voices of his struggling parents persist inside Sam's psyche—it's as though he never grew up and left their house.

Sam's critical inner voice is relentless, demanding that he work hard all the time to "have enough money" and to support the moral imperative to orient to the needs of others first. Unwittingly, Sam has become overidentified with the archetype of the martyr, sacrificing his health and ultimately his life (if he does not change) for others. He is a martyr to his self-devaluing beliefs.

Sam is not an isolated case among high-intensity relaters, who often compromise their self-care. The many common self-sabotaging beliefs that proliferate among high-intensity relaters tend to come with the territory of being an Enneagram personality type Two, the Nurturer (described in Chapter 2). These self-limiting beliefs to orient to the needs of others first often result in Nurturers ignoring the pressing need to retreat, rest, and restore themselves back into homeostasis. In addition, the high levels of sensitivity to outer stimuli that characterize the Highly Sensitive Person temperament (also described in Chapter 2) can exacerbate the self-limiting beliefs to attend to the needs of others first.

High-intensity relaters are generally kind, compassionate and good people who truly want to help the world by helping others in direct service applications. But their unwillingness or inability to say NO to the needs of others because of their underlying beliefs and negative thinking patterns creates the most insidious and persistent self-sabotage. These all too frequent, pervasive personal blocks prevent people from changing in the ways they desire. And when this continues to influence high-intensity relaters, burnout becomes close to inevitable.

However, these personal blocks can be overcome. The following section outlines a strategy that will support you and enable you to succeed.

Silence the inner critic and eradicate self-limiting beliefs

When you feel discouraged or defeated before you even begin something, your observer must have fallen asleep. Its lack of vigilance has made it possible for your inner critic to come to the fore, and for your self-limiting beliefs to convince you that there's nothing you can do to improve your situation. You are likely awash in a wave of neuropeptide stress chemicals. Your opportunity to prevent the critic from intruding into your thoughts has slipped by, and your self-limiting beliefs are preventing you from seeing that there *are* opportunities for you to make positive changes in your situation. What you need is a reliable strategy to confront and quiet down the inner critic and self-defeating beliefs to minimize their negative effect on you.

What works consistently well with my clients is a strategy that I call "stalking the critic." You must assert your own authority and dominion over this negative, seemingly autonomous inner voice by talking back to it—tell it to STOP! This will firmly establish that *you* are the one in control of your thinking process, not your critic. Your approach must be one of asserting yourself in a confrontational way, rather than engaging in any kind of dialogue or pleading with the critic to stop. There can be no negotiation with the critic! Some commentators of the voice dialogue technique argue that there is always value in engaging and trying to understand the motives of the critic (as just another inner part of us demanding our attention). I disagree. There is a distinction to be made between constructive criticism that helps us to learn and improve, and shame-based criticism intended to put us down and diminish us as a person of lesser value. My long experience reflects that, ultimately, the critic must be silenced to allow your mind to gradually expand and become quieter, which is what you need to support your growing awareness that your critic figure is dismissive and devaluing. The critic simply must be quieted and stopped.

As mentioned earlier, an active inner critic is very often an internalized negative parent. If as a child you were not allowed to have a voice to say NO as a way to protect yourself, you may find it very challenging to muster the personal power or the language to speak up assertively and confront your parental legacy. So, in addition to telling that negative voice STOP!, it is helpful to fan the area in front of your solar plexus (that is, in front of your stomach) with one hand, a few inches

> The critic simply must be quieted and stopped.

away from the body. As you do this, say out loud to yourself, "I am the one in charge of this change process and I will prevail over this condemning and judgmental inner voice." You might also add, "Though I couldn't stop the voice when I was a child, I *can* stop this voice now. This voice is just an old thinking habit that I now have control over."

This fanning technique is effective because the solar plexus area is one of the seven major chakras in Indian yogic practices. (The chakras are the centers of our vital energy. Healers from the Indian tradition use the chakras to recruit and regulate our vital energy for healing and balance. For a more comprehensive explanation of the chakras and meridians, you can refer to my first book, *Dynamic Energetic Healing*®.) Specifically, the chakra located in the solar plexus area is associated with challenges related to personal power. As the solar plexus chakra is fanned, unbalanced and contracted vital energy that is directly related to submission and feelings of shame and disempowerment is expanded. This changes the relative balance of the chakras in your body and creates a new energetic configuration. This is a powerful complement to the suggestions above for confronting the disparaging inner voice of the critic.

A very effective complementary approach to asserting your power over your inner critic is to keep a journal. Many people don't realize how dominant and relentless their inner critic is until they develop the habit of journaling at least once a day, preferably in the evening. Journaling helps you reflect on the themes and recurring events that persisted in your awareness that day. Often, journaling helps you to recognize that your childhood experiences in your family of origin are the source of your

> Journaling helps you reflect on the themes and recurring events that persisted in your awareness during that day.

current suffering or feelings of defeat and inadequacy. While this sounds like a stereotypical refrain from traditional psychotherapy, sadly, it remains as true today as it ever was. Sometimes, these feelings are restimulated by a critical or judgmental person in your current work or home life. Some people who journal daily are shocked to discover and acknowledge just how long they have been tyrannized by this under-the-radar habitual thinking pattern that constantly erodes their sense of value and competence. This is often a reflection of having critical, judgmental parents who had their own unhealed traumas.

Note that the strategies described above must be done every day as a regular practice until you begin to notice that your interior mental dissonance becomes quiet and your inner critical voice has receded into the background. This *will* happen as you persist, and you will find that your previously very cluttered negative mental environment will open up to enormous inner spaciousness and quietude.

Is it realistic to expect to tame your inner critic? With conscious intent and a clear understanding of the inner dynamics of your critic process, I assure you that the critic and the accompanying self-devaluing thoughts will wane and eventually lose their sway over you. The ultimate result is great freedom to choose how you want to run your life without the sabotaging influence of old thought patterns. Self-care then becomes *your* choice and your new way of life.

Establishing an inner observer, limiting the inner critic's intrusive negative chatter by telling it to STOP!, and journaling nightly are part of your commitment to self-care. When you make these practices part of your everyday life, you will notice a growing feeling of self-empowerment as you stop the critic from sabotaging your thoughts, health, and outlook.

It is important to note that we all encounter external critics as well as the one inside ourselves. The negative voice can come from another person who is unsupportive, judgmental, jealous or competitive. Learning how to protect yourself from being sabotaged by negative people is discussed in Chapter 7.

Psychoenergetic reversal

Psychoenergetic reversal is another phenomenon that causes people to unwittingly sabotage themselves and their most important self-care goals. Have you ever wondered why it is so difficult for some people to lose weight or exercise regularly when they know they should and want to? From an energy psychology perspective, the concept of psychoenergetic reversal explains how this occurs and what perpetuates their self-sabotaging behaviors.

Briefly, the idea of psychoenergetic reversal was developed by Dr. Roger Callahan, the developer of *Thought Field Therapy*® and one of the early pioneers in the energy psychology field. Callahan called this phenomenon *psychological reversal*.[4] However, since then our knowledge and understanding of energy psychology has grown, and it is now apparent that our vital energy system is integrally associated with this self-sabotaging inner block. Therefore, I believe that the term *psychoenergetic reversal* more accurately defines the phenomenon.

There are a variety of theoretical explanations about what psychoenergetic reversal is, but in simplest terms, you are psychoenergetically reversed when your actions are in conflict with your conscious, intentional desires. If you want to achieve a particular goal or make a positive change in a certain situation or context, and yet the universe at large continues to thwart this conscious intention, take pause to assess what is amiss in your daily efforts. Frequently, psychoenergetic reversal is a primary underlying causative factor.

It is important to note that psychoenergetic reversal can affect almost any aspect of a person's life. Someone who has a conscious desire to excel at a given sport and yet somehow never finds the time to train and practice may be psychoenergetically reversed athletically. A student who has a conscious desire to get good enough grades to be admitted to graduate school and yet doesn't focus enough energy on her studies may be psychoenergetically

> Psychoenergetic reversal can affect almost any aspect of a person's life.

reversed academically. A single person who has a conscious desire to expand his social circle yet never makes the time to meet new people may be psychoenergetically reversed socially. Psychoenergetic reversal can also affect someone's professional life. For example, let's consider the case of Susan.

Susan

Susan is a hospice worker who wants to reduce her workload by ten hours a week so she can spend more time with her two young children. Though financial concerns do not factor into her decision-making process, Susan continues to generate excuses and reasons for why reducing her working hours is not possible. Objectively, her desire to modify her work schedule is certainly possible and desirable, and her decision to continue dedicating those additional ten hours a week to supporting her suffering clients is in direct conflict with what she really wants to do for herself. This is a classic example of someone who may be psychoenergetically reversed. If Susan is psychoenergetically reversed, she will continue to actively sabotage her precious time with her children. She knows they are more important than those ten hours at work, and yet she cannot bring herself to cut her hours. Somehow, she has rationalized the conflict between her behavior and her beliefs.

Many in the energy psychology community theorize that, at a fundamental level, inner conflicts such as Susan's are generated by a reversal of her vital energy flow in relationship to one or more specific underlying beliefs. The theory states that such a reversal is what causes the incongruence between the person's thoughts and actions.

It is likely that psychoenergetic reversal occurs because of long-term conditioning or negative reinforcement about a specific area of your life. This part of your life has been continually and persistently devalued over time and accompanied by a series of associated negative beliefs. In Susan's case, a number of factors conspired to create this psychoenergetic reversal. First, Susan acknowledges that she is definitely an Enneagram Nurturer and is extremely empathic. Thus, her general orientation is first to the needs of others who are in pain, and she literally feels their pain. Another significant factor is Susan's heightened psychic abilities. As she was growing up, her parents and some of her friends teased and criticized her for talking about her experiences with her "imaginary friends," to the point that Susan stopped talking about them. As she became older, she decided that she would tell no one about her unusual perceptions but find ways to help others using her unique abilities. These decisions shaped her beliefs and career direction.

Now, as an adult, she claims to see the spirits of people as they near death, and the guides who are hovering around them to help them make the transition from this life to what is next on their journey. Over many years, Susan has come to realize that if she is present when one of her clients dies, she can communicate with that person's guides and ensure that the person's spirit is supported in a way that she believes ensures their safe passage or transition to the next step in their spiritual evolution. Because she fears for the safety (spiritually speaking) of her dying clients, she is not allowing herself to spend the ten hours per week with her children even though she has a strong desire to do so. She believes that her presence is absolutely necessary for the safe transition of her clients from this world to the next.

Thus, Susan is deeply conflicted. Her conscious intention to spend more time with her children is being eclipsed by her strong feelings of duty toward her clients because she can help them in ways that others cannot. Objectively, she realizes that she cannot realistically be there for everyone who is dying, but her belief is so strong that it has caused her psychoenergetic reversal. She wants to reduce her work hours, yet she cannot bring herself to do it.

This is an example of how a deeply entrenched, habitual belief can become internalized at the subconscious level, perpetuating a disruption and imbalance in your energy system. As a consequence, you end up habitually thinking about yourself in ways that push against what you truly want to do.

Correct the reversal

You could choose to pursue a course of in-depth psychotherapy in order to identify the possible causes of your psychoenergetic reversal or self-sabotage. However, I have learned that in energy psychology applications in general, and psychoenergetic reversal in particular, it is frequently not necessary to understand the underlying reasons for the reversal. It is only necessary that you acknowledge and realize that you continue to be thwarted in your efforts to accomplish a specific goal.

From my experience of working with this issue with many hundreds of clients over the last fourteen years, I've adopted a simple and reliable strategy that is frequently used among energy psychology practitioners to help you achieve what I call whole system congruence. When your whole system is congruent, it means that your conscious self-care intention and your subconscious beliefs are all lined up properly. When this occurs, the unimpeded flow of your vital energy reflects coherence throughout your entire being.

The strategy to achieve whole system congruence is very straightforward. It involves tapping on the side of either hand (known as the "karate-chop" point, which is the small intestine-3 acupuncture meridian point in the middle of the fleshy part of the side of your hand) while repeating the following statement: "I completely and profoundly accept myself, even though I [have this particular problem]." In Susan's case, the entire statement would be "I completely and profoundly accept myself, even though I am conflicted and do not have the resolve to cut back my work schedule by ten hours per week in order to spend more time with my children." Similar set-up statements are, for example, "I completely and profoundly accept myself even though . . .

- I cannot let go of my anger toward my spouse."
- my cravings for chipotle-flavored potato chips are out of control."
- my compulsion to read past midnight prevents me from sleeping through the night."

Repeat your statement out loud three times while tapping the side of one of your hands continuously. It has been empirically determined that the time required to repeat such a statement three times is approximately the time needed to begin to reset your vital energy system in relationship to any thoughts of resistance. Immediately follow this step by *visualizing* yourself achieving your goal and *feeling* relieved and happy to be doing what you desire but were previously unable to do. Spend two to three minutes imagining yourself successfully achieving your desired intention in a variety of contexts and/or with a number of different people.

Frequently, one treatment is enough to successfully treat psychoenergetic reversal pertaining to a specific goal. But there are times when it takes repeated application to permanently correct psychoenergetic reversal related to a specific goal that still remains unrealized.

Although you cannot know for certain that you are psychoenergetically reversed when you start to work on a specific problem, using this technique will tend to neutralize *any* self-defeating and discouraging negative thinking that is sabotaging your efforts, whether the thoughts are in your conscious awareness or have become subconscious over time. This simple approach will reduce any self-sabotaging tendencies that are preventing you from achieving a successful outcome. How will you know if you have been successful in correcting the reversal? When you are able to move forward in action with your desired goals or intentions and continue to follow through to achieve your personal objective.

We are all creatures of habit, and so it is not surprising that we aren't able to make positive changes in our lives instantly. First, we must overcome our old, deeply instilled thinking patterns that shape us even though we may not be consciously aware of them. When you feel that your inner critic, your self-limiting beliefs, psychoenergetic reversal, or some combination of these three phenomena may be holding you back, use the techniques outlined in this chapter to regain control of your thoughts and bring yourself back to a state of whole system congruence. If your situation is a complex one that involves more than one of the phenomena discussed in this chapter, you may find it necessary to use a combination of the techniques discussed to completely eliminate the factors that are holding you back.

> The important thing to remember is that you *can* make positive changes in your life.

The important thing to remember is that you *can* make positive changes in your life. As a high-intensity relater, it is absolutely essential that you honor your own needs and strive to actualize them so that you are at your very best while working with clients and even after your workday is finished. Your well-being is paramount—take yourself seriously.

Questions and Exercises

1. As you daydream about how wonderful it would be to realize a high priority personal or professional goal, pay attention to any doubts that emerge. What is that critical or doubting inner voice saying? Is the tone sarcastic, devaluing or belittling? For example, if your self-care plan involves more travel for occasional personal retreats, do you hear any inner chatter about spending too much money or not having enough time? Make a commitment right now to journal regularly, which will help you identify any repeating themes coming from that inner critical voice. It won't take long before you'll be able to confront that inner critic and, ultimately, shut it down.

2. Do you think you could create an inner observer that watches and listens in on all of your thoughts and activities, especially when you are by yourself? Experiment for a few days to determine if you can do it. An inner observer will help you identify any persisting or underlying self-limiting beliefs that could be contributing to your self-sabotage.

3. Do you live with someone who is frequently critical or judgmental of you? How do you deal with them? Are you able to voice your objections to being put down or verbally abused? Is this enough to stop the criticism? If you do live with a critic figure, assess how much this negative influence may be contributing to your self-sabotage.

4. Do you ever feel that you stop or block yourself from achieving or accomplishing personal goals that are important to you? Does this happen in only one area of your life, or in many? Have you tried several times to achieve these goals, only to be thwarted? If so, you may be psychoenergetically reversed. Consider using the self-care tool described in this chapter as a way to move beyond your stuckness.

CHAPTER

7

The Primary Directive:
Always Take Care of Yourself First

How solid are your energetic boundaries?

In Chapter 2, we looked at the four major models that describe the "helper personality." These models identify the characteristics of individuals who are highly empathic—in other words, individuals who are high-intensity relaters. The common thread that weaves its way through all these personality types and temperaments is the issue of boundaries.

A boundary is a limit that we intentionally establish to protect the integrity of our self and our life. Energetic boundaries keep us connected to ourselves so we can decide what energy, thoughts, and emotions to let in and what to keep out. As I described in my first book, energetic boundaries reframe how we are related to something or someone. Boundaries are not about isolating ourselves by creating a barrier of protection. Rather, boundaries are energetic strategies we use to establish harmony with another context.

> Energetic boundaries reframe how we are related to something or someone.

Consider these examples of weak boundaries:

- If you become depressed in the winter because the weather is cold and dreary, your energetic boundaries with *winter weather* are compromised.

- If you become anxious when you have to give a presentation, your energetic boundaries with *public speaking* are compromised.
- If you find yourself eating healthily during the day but you have a habit of grazing and overeating at home in the evenings, your energetic boundaries are compromised with the specific context of *eating at home in the evenings.*

In contrast, when you have solid and intact energetic boundaries with a context or with another person, you are in optimal appropriate relationship—in harmony—with that "other." Having said that, our understanding of harmony must be appreciated as an interior experience that naturally extends itself to other interactional contexts. It is said among the legendary masters of ancient qigong practice that everything we do expends qi (or chi). We know from the empirical evidence of acupuncture and Chinese medicine that

> human beings are infused with and circulating a kind of energy often referred to as the vital life force. There have been various names for this vital life force throughout history and within many different spiritual traditions. This energy is called *prana* in the practice of yoga, *chi* in Chinese medicine, *ki* in the Korean martial-arts traditions, *power* in the shamanic tradition, and the Holy Spirit in the Christian tradition. In spiritual literature, cross-culturally and throughout history, this vital life force has different names that are synonyms for the same thing.[1]

This vital life force needs to be balanced in ways that replenish our chi and restore inner balance and harmony. If we constantly overspend our energy, we will deplete our energetic bank account and end up energetically, physically and emotionally broke. This is why healthy energetic boundaries are so vital in our lives.

William

William has a very demanding job at a state agency, in which he is ultimately responsible to the governor. He oversees several multimillion dollar projects and supervises managers in locations throughout the state. He must manage and review his agency's budget and meet regularly with each manager, making sure that their respective areas are adequately staffed and they are meeting their deadlines. He loves the challenge of his job and enjoys the many people he must meet with.

Yet, William complains about the unending workload and the seemingly endless e-mails that are constantly demanding his immediate attention. Lately, William has complained that he feels so overwhelmed by his e-mails that he must attend to them before he even leaves his house for work in the mornings, after he finally comes home each evening, and during much of his weekends. He is paid well and enjoys the respect of his peers, but he is so stressed out by his overwhelming responsibilities that he cannot sleep well at night. He has had to resort to prescription sleep medication nightly, and he still only sleeps three to five hours per night.

William is not just a manager, analyst and grant writer—he also happens to be a high-intensity relater. His nervous system is constantly so overstimulated that there is no time in his schedule for him to restore and replenish his chi. William's sympathetic nervous system is in a state of relative fight or flight all the time! From the perspective of chi management, his vital life force is always being expended but never being replenished. William does not realize he is burning himself out through his over-enthusiasm and commitment to a challenging job that does not allow him time and space away from its constant demands and excitation. William is on his way to becoming chronically chi depleted. This will eventually compromise his health and well-being at the physical and emotional levels. If William does not give his nervous system a break, he will end up being energetically broke.

As I explained in my previous book,[2] establishing energetic boundaries is essential for maintaining your inner harmony in a given context or when you are with another person, especially if that person is disagreeable or problematic. Establishing proper boundaries is particularly important for caregivers, since we are often in emotionally challenging situations with people who are difficult to deal with in some way, and our highly empathic nature makes us more susceptible to having weak or porous boundaries.

In fact, if there is any one rule that will sustain a caregiver while working to support other people, it is this: Your first priority is to *always take care of yourself* physically, emotionally, spiritually, and in every other way while in relationship to another. Many people claim that this presumes a kind of self-centeredness or even selfishness, and that it flies in the face of service to others. But I cannot emphasize strongly enough that the need to take care of yourself first is a fundamental truth. For high-intensity relaters, this is actualized via proper maintenance of energetic boundaries. While it is particularly important to maintain proper boundaries with your clients, you must also have adequate boundaries in all major contexts in your life so that you are managing your chi consciously and consistently. As you hone your second attention awareness (see Chapter 5), you will become more sensitive to contexts that require you to examine your energetic boundaries and ensure that they are strong.

> Your first priority is to a*lways take care of yourself* physically, emotionally, spiritually, and in every other way.

An integral part of maintaining proper boundaries with others is acknowledging your own needs and making them your priority. Do you first orient to the needs of the other and their expectations of you, or do you attend to your needs first and foremost? If you do the former, then your first reference point is external, or outside yourself. If you do the latter, your first reference point is internal.

For example, a client's habit of almost yelling at you when she talks (due to her aggressive personality) will, over time, tend to agitate and stimulate your sympathetic nervous system. As a high-intensity relater, your level of innate sensitivity may even cause your fight or flight response to become activated, bringing you a host of symptoms ranging from a racing heartbeat to pounding or migraine headaches. If you tend to orient to the needs of others first, you might remind yourself of how important it is to establish and maintain rapport with your client. You might then decide to practice some deep breathing, and resolve to endure your time with this client because you are helping her to do what *she* needs to do (that is, process her feelings and express herself).

> An integral part of maintaining proper boundaries with others is acknowledging your own needs and making them your priority.

While this approach may be commendable, becoming worn down and overstimulated by someone else's unconscious habit of always speaking in a booming voice sets you up to be a martyr, and it is ultimately self-devaluing. To establish and maintain proper energetic boundaries with this individual, you must become consciously aware of how *your* nervous system is reacting in response to this client. When you do this, your internal referencing with second attention awareness informs you that *you must do something* to create a mutually respectful therapeutic context with this client that is easier for you to manage and more hospitable to you. After all, it is your time and energy you are choosing to spend with this person. By orienting to your own needs in this way (that is, becoming internally focused), you become aware that you must ask this client to speak in a softer voice.

In fact, this intervention is the most compassionate way to help this client, since she probably yells at everyone in her life. Most likely, this is an unconscious defense to keep people at a distance as a way to protect a vulnerable part of her from getting too close and possibly hurt by someone. Ultimately, she ends up alone and disengaged from the people who she would otherwise like to be closer and more connected to. By taking care of yourself in asking her to soften her voice, you are also providing her with an opportunity, in a safe environment, to try out a new way of relating. Over time and with some regular reminders, she will become more available to others to form more meaningful relationships where emotional intimacy becomes possible. But most importantly, by taking care of yourself, you establish reliable energetic boundaries with her as you maintain your integrity within the relational context.

Focusing on external reference points while interacting with another person usually means that you are in denial about your own needs. If this is true of you, you may develop the habit of continually deferring to the needs of others, even when it is to your own detriment. You are in danger of "losing" parts of yourself to the other person. Further, whether you realize it or not, in most circumstances you are complicit in this cumulative loss of self. Your misguided belief systems about (guilt-induced) compassion and selflessness, which are reinforced by a variety of cultural and religious influences, have resulted in you actually giving away parts of yourself.

For example, the young woman who feels bullied into moving in with her boyfriend despite her own misgivings gives away the part of herself that wants to maintain her personal autonomy and be independent. She has given away that inner part of her that knows how to and wants to say NO to others, that is, the part of herself that would allow her to maintain her own integrity. Instead, she continues to orient to the needs of other people first (her boyfriend, in this case) to avoid a possible conflict. This theme tends to repeat itself in many different types of relationships across the spectrum of the population. William, in the example above, gave up to his job the part of himself that needs time alone to reflect and restore himself. While he wasn't exactly being bullied by anyone, he lost his way and became suffocatingly engulfed by the demands of his job. He suffered soul loss, as did the young woman who consented against her better judgment to move in with her boyfriend. These parts of our vital essence are essential for maintaining wholeness and self-integrity. Losing sight of our self-care needs becomes a diminution of our self and of the values that we esteem more than anything else. These values have developed over many years through countless experiences and have become our core self. Devaluing any part of our core essence results in serious compromises to our well-being.

People who habitually give away parts of themselves are called "people pleasers" or "rescuers." Dr. Anne Wilson Schaef was one of the first to write about this in her book *Co-Dependence: Misunderstood—Mistreated.*[3] Schaef and others have discovered that external referencing is the central characteristic that defines the co-dependent personality. Schaef summarizes this well:

> Devaluing any part of our core essence results in serious compromises to our well-being.

> Co-dependents have no concept of a self that others could relate to; whatever small vestige of the self does exist is easily given away in order to maintain a relationship because they feel like literally nothing without the relationship.[4]

Schaef's concept of co-dependency emerged from the alcohol and chemical dependency model, as an elaboration of her understanding of the disease of addiction. However, other theorists have pointed out that the co-dependent personality is a modern cultural archetype. It is frequently reinforced in dysfunctional families, our conformist educational system, and the traditional hierarchical church and religious systems. It is even reinforced by the corporate cultures of many Fortune 500 companies, in which individuality and personal innovation are frowned upon in favor of compliance and conformity to the company's norms and expectations. From all of these systemic influences, many children grow up trained to defer to outer authority. Sadly, in the process they lose touch with their true inner core. As Schaef succinctly puts it,

> Co-dependence is a frightening state of existence. Co-dependents cannot do what they want to do because they have grown so out of touch with their feelings that they cannot determine what it is they even want.[5]

Maintaining our health and well-being demands a commitment to behaviors and practices that reflect our knowledge of what we need to do in order to stay healthy. As your second attention awareness increases, you learn to perceive subtle informational cues that either come from inside yourself (for example, "I am suddenly aware of a *feeling* of general contraction when my client begins talking about his partner"), or that come from an external reference point (for example, "I notice when my client goes on and on in answer to my question about whether he is secure about his relationship to alcohol"). As you become more sensitized to and aware of internal and external referential cues, your ability to maintain energetic boundaries increases, enabling you to say NO when you really mean to, instead of deferring to others' wishes.

Second attention awareness is a skill that you will develop over time as you practice orienting to and staying consciously aware of what is going on within your own thoughts, perceptions, feelings and sensations in relation to your enlarged field of interaction. It is not enough to simply pay attention to the narrative of the person you are attending to—you must also pay attention to what *you* are experiencing as you listen to the person you are helping. If you are receiving double signals, your second attention awareness will allow you to notice your inner confusion and a sense of cognitive dissonance that something is not adding up. As you continue to pay more attention to your experience, you may begin to notice that you are alternating between feeling confused and irritated. If you stay with your experience, you may begin to realize that the person talking to you is so uncomfortable that he is covering up his true feelings. These subtle cues will provide you with important information, as long as you stay with your experience through your second attention awareness. Becoming more internally focused will help you to know the truth and support you in being more compassionate through your deepening understanding.

The importance of saying NO

Most caregivers are confronted daily with a workload and responsibilities that seem to be never ending. There is always another bill to pay, another load of laundry to wash, another treatment plan to prepare and another need to attend to. How is it humanly possible (let alone practical) to replenish ourselves so that we have sufficient stores of chi to maintain the basic raw energy we need for our emotional well-being and physical health? Although it may seem oversimplified, a powerful way to assert healthy boundaries is to say NO often!

For many people, saying NO while they were growing up tended to create conflict with parents or siblings, and these people may have trained themselves not to say it in order to avoid being hurt or abused, and to maintain peace in the family. But it is essential to learn this interpersonal skill in order to maintain proper boundaries with the people who you are attending to. When a person takes on the role of caregiver or helper to another, there is always a contract that deals with mutual expectations and obligations. In professional settings, the contract is formalized; in family caregiving situations, its terms are often unspoken or implied at best. But since boundary issues so often become blurred in the caregiving context, these terms need to be made explicit.

Reflecting on the practice to *consciously* say YES or NO to people (or perhaps taking some time to think about how you genuinely feel before responding) is essential to maintaining healthy and appropriate interpersonal boundaries. This conscious reflection ensures that you are referencing internally, and thus considering your own needs first. From here, appropriate action will naturally follow, whether that means agreeing or saying NO with conviction.

> Reflecting on the practice to *consciously* say YES or NO to people (or perhaps taking some time to think about how you genuinely feel before responding) is essential to maintaining healthy and appropriate interpersonal boundaries.

Saying NO and maintaining excellent boundaries applies beyond the context of the challenges you face when dealing with the person you are caring for. This essential self-care imperative extends to all varieties of interpersonal situations, including those with your boss, co-workers, other family members (including your pets!), and anyone else who makes demands on you. You also need to establish boundaries with time, the media, and your own propensities toward self-destructive behaviors.

We begin by looking at the challenges we face in establishing boundaries with other people.

Boundaries with other people

People who grew up in a dysfunctional family in which their physical and emotional boundaries were never respected often find it difficult to maintain good interpersonal boundaries with people in their adult life. When people have been mistreated or abused, their unconscious adaptive strategy for protecting themselves from being hurt again is to become defended. In a defended state, people are wary and suspicious of others. Sadly, these individuals have great difficulty trusting anyone, because their defenses get in the way of maintaining any kind of mutually respectful ongoing relationship. Common defended behaviors (or defenses) include quiet withdrawal, frequent distrust of others' motives, and little or no self-disclosure. More aggressive defensive behaviors include habitual criticism, outright hostility, and dangerous verbal and physical attacks. When people have not worked on themselves sufficiently to identify and disable their defenses, healthy relationships are simply not possible.

It may surprise you to learn that defensive behaviors are particularly prevalent in helping relationships. Since most of us have not yet completely worked through our personal history and emotional wounding, we unconsciously tend to draw into our lives people who are significantly defended. Issues you haven't yet worked out with your family of origin (in terms of your own wounding) tend to be recreated with people who are drawn into your life to give you a second chance to restore and reclaim the power that was taken from you when you were younger.

Thus, it is common for helpers and caregivers to be in relationships in which they are violated time after time. Some clients may behave angrily toward you, others may try to induce guilt feelings in you, and others may try, perhaps unconsciously, to manipulate your feelings in some other way. Your job as a helper is to be supportive and nonjudgmental in order to help these people deal with their limitations and hopefully grow beyond them. And while you may know, in theory, what to do in order to take care of yourself when dealing with negative, demanding and/or hostile people, putting that knowledge into practice is often surprisingly difficult.

> It is common for helpers and caregivers to be in relationships in which they are violated time after time.

Feeling depleted or drained after a session with one of these clients is caused by more than just an expenditure of your energy. As I explained in the discussion on psychotoxic energy in Chapter 1, information is being exchanged between you and your clients energetically every time you have an interaction. This energetic information can be either supportive or damaging. Though you may not be able to put your finger on it immediately, you probably recognize that some people feel nurturing, life-affirming and supportive to you, while others can be very draining, negative and even hostile.

In reality, some people are just toxic to you—they emanate psychotoxic thoughts and energy. As a highly empathic caregiver, you may recognize that much of that psychotoxicity is being generated from the wounded part in them that was created by unhealed trauma—the part that created their defenses—and that they are likely not consciously aware that they are radiating toxic energy. Knowing this may make you feel even more empathic toward that person, and more determined to help them in any way you can. But you must be alert to protecting yourself from being violated in their presence. *Strong interpersonal boundaries are essential in order to preserve your health and personal well-being.*

> *Strong interpersonal boundaries are essential in order to preserve your health and personal well-being.*

Before we go any further, I would like to look more closely at some of the types of people who challenge us the most to maintain our energetic boundaries and thus our personal integrity.

Energy vampires, drama queens and chaos junkies

In literature and the media, the vampire archetype has become increasingly popular since Bram Stoker wrote *Dracula* in 1897. This vampire myth has popularized the themes of sustaining eternal life via seductive and erotic sucking and draining of blood from the victim. This archetypal interpersonal dynamic can be viewed as a metaphor for a variety of contemporary perpetrator/victim relationships. Directly relevant for us is Dr. Judith Orloff's description of "energy vampires":

> What is common to all vampires is that they take our energy and exhaust us . . . How do you know if you've

encountered a vampire? Even after a brief contact you
leave feeling worse, but he or she seems more alive . . .
It's about being drained when energy is taken from you.[6]

One example of an energy vampire is the person who conveys
to you that he is a total victim and reminds you over and over
again that he has no personal resources to survive emotionally in
the world without you. This person is needy, dependent and always
complaining. You can become easily seduced by this energy vampire
because no matter how hard you try to support him, nothing ever
changes. For a caregiver, this situation is a self-defeating setup to
try harder and compromise your boundaries until you find yourself
available to this person not only during his appointment times but
throughout your busy day and even after hours when his pleading
phone calls or e-mails ask for your help. When working with this
type of personality, it is easy to get in over your head by putting in
extra hours and becoming preoccupied with the person's misery
and never-ending problems, which he constantly reminds you of.
If you are not able to recognize this energy vampire from the
beginning, your vital essence will slowly and progressively be
depleted, just like the classic Dracula victim. In order to maintain
your own vital energy and be able to replenish yourself, you must
set limits with the amount of time you are willing to spend interacting with this energy vampire.

A particular type of energy vampire is what Orloff calls the
"drama queen"[7] and what I call the "chaos junkie" or "Mr./Ms
Extreme States." The drama queen has no interest in what you are
feeling. He or she controls the relationship with intense, out-of-
proportion emotionality and increasing volume. Screaming and
crying accompany wide fluctuations in mood, from extreme self-
pity to anger and rage. As the caregiver intent on supporting this
individual, you are most likely in a constant state of startle.
Exhausted and drained after being with this person for thirty to
sixty minutes, you wonder what you can do the next time to help

calm them down so they will take in your suggestions on how to gain more self-control.

Frequently, chaos junkies are narcissistic, insensitive and unrestrained. An inherent problem with these vampires is that when they are in their extreme state, nobody is home to mediate the emotional excess. This means that by necessity your tasks become trying to survive the raging storm that erupts out of nowhere, intervening during the occasional calm, and anticipating the next tempest that blows through your energy field. Ms. Extreme States cannot help herself, so you are constantly under attack. Your symptoms may be varied and unique to your own sensibilities, but symptoms you will have—perhaps a migraine starts in the middle of an encounter, or you get that queasy feeling that means you're about to be sick from creeping anxiety that continues to grow. You may even experience the spacey feeling that comes when you start to leave your body.

Falling into old co-dependent tendencies with this energy vampire will not only be draining, it will ultimately be physically deleterious and destructive to your life. Chaos junkies thrive on their extreme states while draining your life force in an interpersonal energetic vortex that finds you flailing and eventually sinking.

Critics and judges

Another of the many varieties of energy vampires is the critic or judge. Known by many names, the critic is not interested in a mutually supportive relationship. He or she is constantly scrutinizing you, always managing to find fault in whatever you do to try to be helpful. He blames and judges, leaving no openness for discussion. Over time, a sincere helper or caregiver gets worn down and begins to feel downtrodden. No matter what you say or do, the critic attacks you without regard to your feelings. For all your skills and compassion, you end up feeling that you are never good enough.

We are inherently vulnerable to this type of energy vampire for a plethora of reasons. One of the main factors that makes many people vulnerable is that they grew up in a family in which they were criticized as part of the family culture. This is an intergenerational problem that is pandemic in most dysfunctional family systems. These children often grow up feeling "not okay" in all kinds of ways: not smart enough, not attractive enough, not athletic enough, and on it goes. In fact, this is a major reason that people end up in therapy—they do not feel connected to others because as children they had to create defenses to protect themselves from the onslaught of constant blame and judgment. They learned to shield themselves from getting too close to others, lest they open themselves to another attack. Meanwhile, their self-esteem was eroded by their critical parent(s). Their feelings of guilt and shame became deeply imprinted in their unconscious sense of self, because their internalized wounded child part stays locked in relationship with the blaming, critical parent. When these children grow up and leave their family, they internalize the critical parent and carry the wounding of the vulnerable inner child with them. When they find themselves in relationship with an intimate other or with a client they are trying to support, it is often the case that the critic ends up sitting across from them.

The caregiver's vulnerable inner child and the critic/judge are inextricably linked in a way that drains the life force from the caregiver. Unless the caregiver has worked out his or her own victim/child–persecutor/critical parent inner dynamic in therapy, he or she usually ends up feeling guilty, insufficient and progressively drained by the accusations and judgments voiced by their client (or aging parent). The critical onslaught overwhelms the caregiver's goodwill, and unless the person being criticized is able to establish proper boundaries with the critical one, the relationship will become destructive and ultimately end in dissolution.

How to protect yourself from energy vampires

Step 1: *Learn to identify them*

While it is easy to spot some energy vampires (such as a person who regularly blames or criticizes you), this archetype has many dimensions to it. Frequently, this energy vampire initially appears charming, intelligent and well organized. Because of a tendency toward perfectionism, these vampires often present themselves as well put together and informed. It is surprising how sure they are of themselves—they pronounce their judgments as if there could be no other reasonable choice. Initially, these features tend to obscure who is really there in front of you. Many caregivers and helpers, who often perceive things in shades of nuance because of their high interpersonal intelligence, are actually drawn to these critic figures, who appear to know a lot and have little doubt. Their disguise may fool you at first, but you will gradually discover that your opinions matter little, and that their opinions gradually transform into condemnatory and judgmental criticism of who you are and what you do. When you begin to feel belittled and dismissed, you will know you are dealing with this vampire. It is surprising how easily a well-disguised energy vampire can blindside you and drain your energy.

How do you know when you have been interacting with an energy vampire? Check in with your body to find out how it is doing.

- Are your muscles comfortable and relaxed?
- Is your breathing constant and regulated?
- Is your heart beat normal?
- Is your posture open?
- Are you feeling in rapport and in synch with the person sitting across from you?

If you answer *yes* to these questions, these primarily somatic feedback cues are informing you that the person you are interacting with is *not* running over or violating your energetic boundaries.

In this situation, you are feeling emotionally safe, and thus you can more easily radiate compassion from a caring, attentive place.

On the other hand, if you answer *no* to the above questions, you are probably feeling disempowered and physically depleted. In this situation, it becomes imperative that you use conscious self-care strategies. In the context of interacting with an energy vampire, this means setting and maintaining consistent limits, including limits on how much time you spend with the person.

Step 2: *Recheck your boundaries*
To prevent being contaminated by a vampire's negative energy, you must exercise clear and sustainable boundaries. Here are some helpful approaches:

- Make sure you take an occasional time-out to reorient from the chaos junkie or judging client and bring your focus back within yourself. It is usually best to leave the environment temporarily, by saying, for example, "I have to use the bathroom for a moment." Doing this breaks the interpersonal trance and allows you to regroup to prevent your nervous system from becoming overloaded.
- Visualizing a protective shield of white light enveloping you can be surprisingly helpful in warding off, deflecting and insulating you from a vampire's verbal attacks or extreme states. (For more on visualization, see Chapter 11.)
- As discussed above, use the general boundary-strengthening tactic of saying NO, which establishes limits on the other person's behavior that is negatively affecting you. It is sometimes necessary to communicate how other people's behaviors affect you to provide them with information and feedback. For example, "I don't like the way you are talking to me right now. It feels attacking." Or, use the well-known "I message" approach; for example, "When you criticize and blame me, I feel defensive and become aware that I want to move further away from you." Saying NO to energy vampires gives

them a chance to re-evaluate whether they are willing to modify their behavior in order to stay in the relationship.

- If your requests to stop the blaming, criticizing and judging continue to be ignored, you may have to create a physical boundary by severely limiting the time you spend with this person.

Step 3: *Know your limits*

As a caregiver, you need to know your own limitations. You will not be able to help everyone who comes to you for help. When you realize that you are unable to maintain strong, protective boundaries, or that you are beyond your capacity to be an effective helper (that is, you feel that you're in way over your head), actually leaving the relationship may be the only way to protect yourself.

For example, if you find yourself trying to downplay or minimize your client's trauma, or changing the subject when the client's graphic and detailed account becomes particularly distressing, this may be a sign that you are experiencing secondary traumatization (see Chapter 1). Anna Baranowsky calls this the silencing response. You cannot be fully present for your client if his or her experience is simply too overwhelming for you to deal with.[8] Another indication that you may need to sever the relationship is when hearing a client's traumatic story makes you question your own beliefs about the world being a safe place. In both of these examples, your emotional overwhelm is indicative of your unhealed personal trauma, compassion fatigue and potential burnout. This is sometimes referred to as countertransference and may indicate that you need to do some of your own therapy to depotentiate your unhealed

> If your requests to stop the blaming, criticizing and judging continue to be ignored, you may have to create a physical boundary by severely limiting the time you spend with this person.

trauma in order to continue working effectively with clients who bring in their own unhealed traumatic residue.[9]

If you are experiencing this type of countertransference, you need to either seek trauma reduction therapy for yourself or sever your relationship with this client entirely by referring the client to another caregiver who is better able to work with him or her. However, I realize that if you are a caregiver for a family member or friend, you may think you cannot make a referral because you're the only one who can help them. Please remember that your first priority is to protect yourself from being violated by the person and *always take care of yourself.* Don't let your limiting belief that you have no way to remove yourself from your involvement with this person set you on the path to self-destruction. If you are willing to acknowledge that everyone—including you—needs and is worthy of receiving help, you will find the strength to seek out the support that you need.

> Don't let your limiting belief that you have no way to remove yourself from your involvement with this person set you on the path to self-destruction.

If you do not proactively take yourself out of a violating situation, it is likely that you will become progressively more traumatized and find yourself losing your health, resiliency, energy and, ultimately, your spirit. No doubt you will be confronted with many difficult and problematic people. Staying in your power and being aware of the interpersonal challenges will help you appreciate how important it is to maintain solid energetic boundaries with everyone you are supporting.

Julia

An excellent example of someone dealing with interpersonal boundary issues is Julia, a psychotherapist who came to me for a supervision session. When Julia came to me for help, she had been a practicing clinician for over twenty years. She had become preoccupied with a former client, Paula, who had died six months earlier from Parkinson's disease. Julia kept saying that she should have and could have done more for Paula, and that *she felt responsible in some way for Paula's death*.

Paula's physician had referred her to Julia after the death of Paula's mother. Paula felt very emotionally bonded to her mother, and she had been bereft since her mother's death. Julia interpreted this as extreme emotional neediness and an acute grief response to the loss of a loved one. Paula also suffered from ongoing general anxiety and other post-traumatic stress symptoms (such as insomnia, regular nightmares, and dependence on Xanax to deal with her anxiety).

For reasons that will be revealed shortly, Julia began to lose control of her therapy sessions with Paula. When Paula came in for an appointment, she would talk non-stop and essentially run out the entire hour. For Julia, this created a feeling of professional inadequacy, since Paula's emotional neediness was overrunning Julia's ability to intervene in any kind of structured therapeutic manner. Julia ended up just silently praying for Paula, and essentially doing a lot of active listening.

Julia had never talked to me about this kind of client-related problem in the past, so I wondered what was so different about this situation. Part of it could have been that Julia herself, from a very young age, felt responsible for her own mother's emotional well-being, and had difficulty maintaining emotional separation and healthy energetic boundaries with her. Another factor could have been how dependent Paula had been on her mother, and that Paula was now transferring that dependency onto Julia. Paula often told Julia how important Julia was to her, and how she didn't think that she could survive without her. As time progressed, Paula became an energetic vampire to Julia.

I was not surprised when manual muscle testing indicated that Julia had no energetic boundaries with Paula, even though Paula had died six months prior. Muscle testing also confirmed that Julia began to experience out-of-proportion grief and sadness when Paula died. It is likely that Julia's experience was partly vicarious trauma (see Chapter 1). As discussed earlier, it is an inherent hazard or risk for caregivers (who lack sufficient energetic boundaries) to absorb the trauma of their client or patient.

As I continued muscle testing, it was confirmed that Julia had no energetic boundaries with her client Paula. As a result, Julia had unwittingly opened up her energy field for Paula's spirit to become literally attached to her. In the shamanic paradigm this is considered a very serious condition. Further muscle testing indicated that the best way to release this attached spirit of Julia's previous client would be through a traditional shamanic journey. This is when the shaman or shamanic practitioner enters a light trance state (usually accompanied by a percussive beat generated by a drum or rattle) to seek the assistance of his or her spiritual guides or helpers in resolving the issue.

Julia was familiar with this ancient healing practice, so she unreservedly agreed to this approach. We burned white sage in the office to create "sacred space" and called in our respective spiritual resources to support our healing work. Julia sat quietly with her eyes closed as I began rattling to shift my consciousness into the light trance state of "non-ordinary reality" to begin my shamanic journey. (Other ways of working with your inner guides are discussed in Chapter 11.) In a short time, one of my guides, who refers to herself as Grandmother, appeared. She gathered the women of her tribe around Julia as they began drumming to impart power and protection into Julia. Then Grandmother perceived that Paula's spirit had indeed attached itself to Julia's energy field in the area of her upper back. What was even more surprising was that Paula's mother had become attached to Paula just after her death! As I continued to rattle, Grandmother called forth a large brown bison, which she said was Paula's and her mother's power animal or spirit guide. Grandmother directed the bison to take Paula and her mother to meet their spiritual family so they could move on to their respective spiritual evolution. (I perceived all this in a light trance state.)

Grandmother then imparted wisdom to Julia (through me as Julia's intermediary), telling her that she cannot interfere with someone else's destiny (in this case, Paula's), since we each have our destiny already written in our soul. Grandmother reminded Julia that we all have our limitations and that it is never Julia's responsibility to heal someone else. We can support someone else in their healing process, but we cannot take personal responsibility, since that would be intervening in their destiny.

When we were finished, Julia's muscle testing indicated that she was free and clear of any residual negative influence from Paula. By releasing the energetic influences of Paula and Paula's mother that Julia had allowed to attach to her (through her lack of sufficient energetic boundaries), Julia had spontaneously released all of the residual trauma related to her preoccupation with Paula. We had confirmed that Julia had been experiencing vicarious traumatization—she had absorbed the grief of Paula and Paula's mother and had mistaken it as her own grief because of the complicated relationship she had with her own mother while growing up. Not surprisingly, her muscle testing reflected that she now had 100 percent energetic boundaries with Paula; Julia was no longer carrying any of Paula's energy.

Because Julia has a high degree of empathy and is an Enneagram type Two, the Nurturer, it has been an ongoing challenge for her to maintain energetic separation from Paula and all the rest of her clients.

Julia's experiences with Paula illustrate the challenge for all caregivers that is inherent in the caregiving relationship. This ongoing challenge is to stay completely present with yourself while you feel into the suffering of your clients and, orienting from your heart, maintain a compassionate detachment to avoid falling under the spell of their neediness and getting swallowed up by their pain. In short, the challenge is to maintain your energetic boundaries to protect yourself from "catching" or absorbing negative energy from your clients. Because Julia had been unable to do this, Paula's pain and suffering leaked into her energy field and took up residence there.

Maintaining solid energetic boundaries will keep you from becoming infected by your clients' travails. Easy to do? Absolutely not. But with knowledge and ongoing second attention awareness, you can maintain appropriate energetic boundaries so that you can do your job effectively and stay healthy at the same time.

When your energetic boundaries with other people are strong, you know how to place limits on the defended behaviors or actions of individuals who may hurt you. At the same time, your boundaries still allow into your life people who have proven themselves to be trustworthy and who emanate positive energy, so your friendships with such people develop and flourish. Mutually respectful relationships become possible when two people are willing to be vulnerable and acknowledge their own flaws in order to cultivate trust in an ongoing relationship.

For those of us who, in our professional or personal lives, are supporting someone who is experiencing emotional or physical pain and stress, Grandmother's wisdom bears repeating: We all have our limitations. It is never our responsibility to heal someone else. We can support someone else in their own healing process in a variety of ways, but we cannot take responsibility for our clients. That would be intervening in someone else's destiny, and it would open

> We all have our limitations. It is never our responsibility to heal someone else.

ourselves up too much to having our own life force drained away. In addition to this age-old wisdom, it is extremely important for us to be aware of our own well-being and be willing to value, cherish and optimize it.

Other important boundary contexts for high-intensity relaters

Boundaries with time

Most of us have passively agreed to abide by the societal construct that time is linear. In other words, we have agreed to the constraints placed on us by the societal definition of time. On a day-to-day basis, we are ruled by the clock—we get up at a certain time, go to work at a prescribed time, and are allowed to leave when our scheduled workday is over. This is generally true whether one is a factory worker, a bank teller, a teacher or an electrician. We are also governed by the calendar, which means that most of us work five days a week throughout the year and, if we are lucky, we get two or three weeks of "time off" for vacation. In our society, time is also directly linked to money. We pay other people for their time and their specialized service to us (the plumber who comes to our house and the mechanic who fixes our car), just as we offer specialized services to others in exchange for money. Most of us accept these schedules and their link to time because having a job to make money to pay our bills is something we must do to survive.

Life is short and capricious, so time is very precious. Each of us is the final arbiter of how we expend our vital force in this unique experience that is our life. Ultimately, how much time we spend on any given pursuit is a reflection of how we have prioritized our deepest personal values. *Whether or not you are in the role of helper or caregiver, the way you use your time defines your life.* But as caregivers, we tend to experience more than average tension between being overly generous and selfish with our time, since by nature we try to be as helpful and giving as possible. We allocate significant chunks of our time to support others who need us (and our time), and are often under pressure

> *The way you use your time defines your life.*

to give still more of our time. As a result, we must be especially vigilant about consciously deciding how we use our time. While it may sound selfish, *your highest obligation or priority in your relationship to time is to yourself!* You must establish limits to allocate your time intentionally, and pay extra attention to what you do with your discretionary time.

In the twenty-first century, this can be quite a challenge. It is so easy to lose ourselves in the multitude of seemingly endless and engaging activities that we might characterize as recreational, such as surfing the internet, reading, watching the latest DVDs, and responding to endless e-mails (that are sometimes actually related to our work). When we allow these pursuits to take over large amounts of our time, we can easily lose our impetus to prioritize, and thus we unwittingly lose touch with what we need to replenish ourselves daily. We literally drain our vital life force energy and devalue ourselves when we are not intentional and judicious in our relationship to time. Apple co-founder and creative genius Steve Jobs frequently expressed the impossibility of being all things to all people. Apple's enormous business success came from focusing on quality and innovation with respect to a small ensemble of key products. He said that much of Apple's success

> While it may sound selfish, *your highest obligation or priority in your relationship to time is to yourself!*

> comes from saying no to 1,000 things to make sure we don't get on the wrong track or try to do too much. We're always thinking about new markets we could enter, but it's only by saying no that you can concentrate on the things that are really important.[10]

To maintain proper energetic boundaries with time (so that you stay in your power and are deliberate with your time, even as you stick to your schedule), it is essential to create enough time in your day to nourish and replenish yourself amid all the demands placed on you by work and family. Only you can decide which of your personal needs are most important and inviolable. If you do not make conscious decisions for how you spend your time on a daily basis, someone else will surely make those decisions for you. That is why maintaining firm and consistent energetic boundaries with the people and things that demand your attention and time is essential.

> If you do not make conscious decisions for how you spend your time on a daily basis, someone else will surely make those decisions for you.

Boundaries with the media

The primary context for caregivers is the interpersonal field. As we have seen, dedicated high-intensity relaters are vulnerable to compassion fatigue and secondary traumatization. Consequently, caregivers must be vigilant about focusing on self-regulation and a daily stress management regimen to maximize their ongoing self-care to insulate themselves from burnout-related symptoms. Although many people have never given it much thought, to be effective this self-care must include taking conscious control of our daily relationship to the media.

Following the 9/11 terrorist attacks and the news coverage of hurricanes Katrina and Rita, I had many clients come to my office experiencing media shock and vicarious trauma from listening to and watching the news coverage of these disasters. In every case, clients expressed fears for their own safety and for their future. Without exception, they were significantly dissociated, and many were experiencing acute anxiety with complaints of insomnia and inability to concentrate.

The insistent demands made by the various forms of media pull us toward adopting an externalized focus rather than an internal one. In spite of this, high-intensity relaters must create strategies and practices to ensure self-protection and proper self-care in order to stay healthy and maintain a sense of being in control of their world. Otherwise, the intrusion of the media will slowly seduce you until it becomes an addiction that swallows you up.

Specifically, you must maintain second attention awareness to ensure that your squeezed emotional feelings and physical fatigue do not take you over into some kind of self-medicating albeit temporary solace. Most people think of addiction as being related to a substance, such as alcohol or drugs (whether prescribed or illegally obtained). In these transient drug-induced altered states of consciousness, one's normal capacities to think and feel become overrun by the temporary numbness and alteration of consciousness that the substance provides. Yet there are process addictions that are just as powerful and self-destructive as any generated by substance abuse. Anything powerful enough to hijack our attention and redirect us from our everyday feeling states and the demands of our daily lives can become an addiction—a temporary escape from our everyday world. Ominously, caregivers and helpers are just as vulnerable to this hijack as any other segment of the general population.

While it would be naïve to completely swear off the news to protect yourself from all the sensationalized violence that has become common in newscasts, watching the TV or internet news just before going to bed is not something I would recommend as a way to calm yourself before drifting off into deep and undisturbed sleep after a day of intense emotional relating. Please take note of how you interact with the media. Do you have healthy limits with this potential time sink? If not, you risk the possibility of falling into addiction. More than

> Staying conscious of your relationship with the media will support your healthy energetic boundaries.

anything else these days, the media grab our attention and seduce us with the latest technology to keep us networked and informed.

Staying conscious of your relationship with the media will support your healthy energetic boundaries.

Boundaries with self-destructive behaviors

In order to say YES to all the new ideas and healthy practices for regularly replenishing yourself that make sense to you, you must first train yourself to say NO to all the seductions our culture insists that we participate in.

Until September 2008, spending and purchasing as an activity (i.e., shopping) was the underlying foundation of the zeitgeist of our time. I am referring to the collective hypnotic trance called consumerism ("I must have this!") which, until the 2008 economic meltdown, had become the American preoccupation that met all the criteria of a religious movement. The preachers come through the media, urging us to buy flat-screen televisions, next-generation iPads and smart phones, the newest laptop computers and other, non-technology, "essentials" to ensure that our lifestyle is optimized and we feel good. At the same time, to be successful is to emulate celebrities. Unlike the themes that prevailed in the 1960s and 70s, which emphasized human potential and expanding consciousness, today's media glamorize and exhort us to lifestyles underpinned by excess.

But how "real" is the reality that is portrayed endlessly in the media? In recent years, millions of Americans have had their homes foreclosed. A number of the biggest Wall Street banks were shut down, or barely survived on government bailout money (although now they are flourishing again!). We also now know that many professional baseball players who received multimillion dollar contracts were doping with steroids (I specifically refer to Alex Rodriguez's admission that he took steroids from 2001 to 2003. He won the American League's Most Valuable Player Award in 2003).

I believe that caregivers need to beware of becoming seduced by consumerism and the false goal of the "having it all" lifestyle, which are distractions to self-care. The constant messages we receive about "getting more," "doing more," and "keeping up" are highly stimulating, which makes it even harder for many high-intensity relaters to calm their already-aroused nervous systems. Caregivers need to kick back and rest to restore their chi, not allow themselves to become more agitated. Spending all or most of your discretionary time interacting with "friends" on Facebook is not evil, but it may cut into the time that you would otherwise spend replenishing your chi by exercising, appreciating nature, spending quality time with your family, further educating yourself, or working on more constructive creative projects.

Other threats to our self-care include the temptations of unhealthy foods and recreational drugs. It is difficult to say NO to comfort foods and other substances that temporarily help us to feel more calm and satiated amid the demands placed on us each day, particularly for caring professionals who have shared in their clients' horrific stories of pain, suffering and abuse. Though we may feel that life is just too much at times, in fact it is we who tend to fall into habitual lifestyle excesses that we just accept as the way our lives have to be.

Saying NO to the overindulgences in our lives is not just about our profligate use of food, alcohol, drugs and, increasingly, high-tech gadgets. But just as we must learn to say NO to working too many hours, to energy vampires, and to trivial activities that use up too much of our spare time, we must also become aware of and turn away from any of the self-destructive behaviors that overstimulate our already overaroused nervous systems. These include such things as sitting in front of the computer or our large-screen televisions for countless hours, watching and listening to intense and often violent multimedia entertainment.

As caregivers and helpers continue to be present for those who are in dire need and frequently in significant emotional and physical pain, maintaining proper boundaries with clients becomes an absolute requirement. High-intensity relaters must create and use strategies and practices that will help them stay healthy and maintain a sense of being in control of their world, in spite of the incessant demands coming from all directions to externalize their attentional absorption and focus. You must learn how to weaken the power that toxic individuals, energetic vampires, intrusive media, and self-destructive behaviors have over you as you deal with them every day. Several strategies have been discussed above, as well as in Chapters 5 and 6. In Chapter 8, I focus my discussion on how to protect and care for yourself by staying strong, healthy, empowered and "centered."

> You must learn how to weaken the power that toxic individuals, energetic vampires, intrusive media, and self-destructive behaviors have over you as you deal with them every day.

Questions and Exercises

1. Do you stand up for yourself when you are challenged? Do you say NO when necessary to establish appropriate limits on what others expect of you? Do you do this with clients as well as with your friends and partner?

2. Have you ever acted in a co-dependent manner? Do you now?

3. Imagine that time is just a human construct and ultimately an illusion. Let yourself dream for a moment, seeing yourself accomplishing everything that you wish to accomplish today and every day this week. Decide for yourself right now that time is your ally, always encouraging you to fulfill your most important desires. Start telling yourself that you have all the time you need to accomplish everything that is important in your life. Notice what changes in your inner reality and/or external life as you continue affirming this new belief.

4. Decide for yourself right now that being honest and authentic is how you choose to conduct yourself in all of your relationships. Consider that there is another way to interact with people than just protecting that tender part inside of you. Make a short list of the most important people in your life. Decide that you are going to fully occupy the relationship with each of these individuals. Practice visualizing yourself surrounded by a globe of radiating white or golden light. Imagine interacting with each of these important individuals within your globe of light. Are others positively affected by your light? Feel what it's like to have solid energetic boundaries with others. Consider the possibilities that accompany this kind of worry-free self-confidence.

5. Think about the people who you interact with regularly. Are any of them energy vampires? These energy drainers can deplete your energy and metaphorically leave you to the buzzards. How do you deal with criticizers, blamers or drama queens? How do you protect your vital energy when you are around an energetic vampire? Imagine interacting with any of them from an attitude of placing high value on your self-care. Imagine what it would be like to say "I don't appreciate it when you talk to me that way. It feels disrespectful to me." What might be some of the long-term consequences if you decided to walk away from the interaction, or even leave the relationship altogether? Are you willing to consider this way of relating to others?

6. Think about any deleterious emotional or physical symptoms that you've developed over time. Are you aware that your body may be storing psychotoxic residue from your interactions with energy vampires that is depleting your vital energy? Start paying close attention to your symptoms, continuing to wonder what information they are storing and trying to convey to you.

7. Just for a minute, imagine that you are truly interconnected with all things and that your thoughts positively influence other people all the time. Using your growing understanding of nonlocal intentionality, think about some new and different ways in which your own growing state of self-coherence will affect your clients and loved ones. Here are some questions to think about over the coming days: How long are you willing to experiment with your new intentional thinking on this? Can you maintain this for at least one week? Be curious and notice the feedback you receive. Do you truly want to change? Do you think you can?

8. In general, how well are you currently taking care of yourself? This is a good time to take a few minutes to find out, before you read on to the next chapters. Appendix 2 provides two checklists for you to use to determine your current level of risk of experiencing secondary trauma, burnout and compassion fatigue. Complete the checklists as honestly as you can, and then consider carefully the information in the *What do your results mean?* section. Appendix 2 will help you to become more conscious of your current state of well-being and the effectiveness of your current self-care measures.

CHAPTER

8

Partnering With Plants:
A Return to Our Roots

This chapter is about how the healing properties of plants can be brought into the caregiver's domain for powerful and effective self-care. However, it does much more than simply recommend that you eat your daily portions of fruits and vegetables. In the text that follows, I describe specific ways in which we can renew our connection to the plant world and be supported by it energetically, emotionally and physically, even as we help others to alleviate their own pain and suffering. Moreover, it is about how we can get back to our roots, so to speak, and open ourselves to the healing powers of plants.

Some people marvel at the ability of plants to capture sunlight through photosynthesis and provide us with the energy that sustains all life. They are aware that, from the time when humans were first on Earth until the rise of our recent postindustrial societies, plants played an integral part in our lives as teachers and healers. This was true across widely diverse cultures, regardless of geographic location or time period.

But I believe that the vast majority of modern people, particularly Westerners, give little thought to our relationship to the plant world. As pressures from overpopulation and inequitable or insufficient food supplies steer us toward further industrial mechanization and monoculture production of food (such as corn, rice and soybeans), our personal relationship to the plant world is shifting dramatically.

From a larger ecological perspective, our relationship to the plant world is not just about providing us with the next meal. Rather, it represents a fundamental thread that weaves its way through all cultures and all people. As caregivers and healthcare providers, plants are available to support us daily, even though most of us take the plant world for granted and never even think about it.

Amid the inexorable pace of progress that our technology-driven society forces on us, it is important to reflect on how our larger relatedness to our particular culture and nation—and to the natural world—profoundly affects us every day. While I marvel at the ease with which I can instantly communicate with others all over the world via my cell phone or voice-over-internet programs (such as Skype), I am also aware that I pay a price for this. It is often the case that once logged on to my computer, internet searches and e-mail correspondence rob me of inordinate hours of my valuable time. Like millions of others, I sit in front of an LCD screen for several hours every day, and feel noticeably drained by the time I am finally able to log off.

But I count myself among the lucky ones, because my work demands that I sit face-to-face with people who I come to honor and respect in the sanctity of my therapy office. It is during these sessions with clients that I open myself up to the subtle nuances of interpersonal communication and energetic information fields. I listen attentively and provide a variety of means to assist my clients to recover from and resolve old traumas so that their True Self becomes once more available. Yet, no matter how deeply meaningful and satisfying these interactions are, at times they also leave me feeling tired and even a bit weary by the end of a long day. So, throughout much of the year, when finished with my workday, I look forward to entering the private refuge of my

> Plants are available to support us daily, even though most of us take the plant world for granted and never even think about it.

home gardens, where I enjoy reconnecting with the natural world. I can feel my stores of chi, which I expended with clients during my workday, being replenished.

Our relatedness to plants

I live in the Pacific Northwest, and I add to our rain forest garden every year, populating it with native plants such as rhododendrons, azaleas, salal and wild huckleberry. In both our flower and our vegetable gardens, I have noticed that certain plants do better and thrive in certain locations. I will provide two brief examples.

A number of years ago I planted strawberry starts in one of our raised beds. I fertilized them and watered them, but after four years of unproductive growth, I finally decided to give up on them and return the bed to vegetables. As you may know, strawberries send out runners as a way to expand their colony and reproduce. I had noticed that a few of the strawberry plants had sent out runners and taken root just next door, in our rose garden. Out of curiosity and sympathy to the strawberries, I allowed those newly established runners to remain. It is three years since I gave up on the strawberries in the raised bed, and strawberries have now carpeted our rather large rose garden as if I planted them as a cover crop. This year, we harvested quarts and more quarts of strawberries for a longer period of time throughout the spring and into the summer than we were ever able to do when they were in the raised bed. The innate intelligence of the strawberry plants knew exactly what area of the garden they preferred in order to proliferate and prosper.

I had a similar experience with the huckleberry plants in my backyard. Originally, I intended them to be a hedge along one edge of the garden. After two years of very little growth, I moved two of the plants just outside our dining room window overlooking our backyard. These two plants have absolutely taken off and clearly like their new location, in contrast to the two stunted plants that remain on the edge of the garden.

These examples illustrate that plants are sentient beings that prefer very specific locales to maximize their growth and the dissemination of their seeds. Might it be that the strawberry plants do better in their new location because we give more attention to the rose bushes (and thus the strawberries get more attention as well), as we collect and trim their flowers regularly throughout the spring and summer? Are the huckleberries by the dining room window growing so vigorously because we admire them every morning while having our breakfast? Is the success experienced by these plants associated with an enhanced relatedness to us? Might these plants be a reminder to us all to open ourselves to nurturing environments so we too can be the beneficiaries of positive regard and greater openness to receive loving and healing input? These speculative questions cannot be answered objectively, but I am reminded of what Michael Pollan suggests in his book *In Defense of Food*.

Our relatedness compromised

Pollan's critique of what he calls the quasi-scientific beliefs that make up the ideology of "nutritionism" assails the industrial food system for disrupting the natural, interconnected links that create our food chains. While the health of the soil has been inextricably linked to the health of the plants and animals that come from it (that we end up eating), Pollan observes that the connections among local soils, local foods and the local populace have been permanently disrupted to such a degree that the biochemical requirements of the human body are now being regularly compromised. Additionally,

> Thousands of plant and animal varieties have fallen out
> of commerce in the last century as industrial agriculture
> has focused its attention on the small handful of high
> yielding (and usually patented) varieties, with qualities

that suited them to things like mechanical harvesting and processing.[1]

A nutrient bias is built into the way reductionistic nutrition science extracts single components from complex whole foods and persuades us that processed foods filled with certain vitamins and minerals (that is, chemical compounds) are healthy for us. Meanwhile, we are becoming ever more disassociated from the essential social and ecological relationships that human beings have always been connected to. We are moving away from the sensual or aesthetic enjoyment of our relationship to food within the larger context of family and community, and as we "eat and run," we are moving toward a primarily utilitarian approach to nourishing ourselves with food. This trend diminishes what has always been a reliable and enjoyable ritual of replenishing our vital force through the celebration of good company sharing good food. Renewing our conscious relationship with the enjoyment of good food is a wonderful means of regular self-care that is easier than, for example, a disciplined meditation practice.

Pollan asserts that over the last three decades, the prevailing nutritional advice has, in fact, "left us fatter, sicker, and more poorly nourished."[2] In addition, the endless variety of scientifically researched and recommended diets have left millions of people regularly feeling confused and guilty about the foods they eat, because those foods do not conform to what they believe nutrition science says they should be eating to maintain optimal health. These realities are completely antithetical to optimal physical and emotional self-care management.

The point I want to make is that because of these new trends based on scientific knowledge or this growing ideology known as nutritionism, we are moving further and further away from being in relationship to the foods we eat. As we think less and less about the web of life that comprises the food chains (soils, plants, animals and humankind), we have become less connected to the natural world and the incredible magic that ancient peoples knew is inherent in our interrelatedness.

Our ancestors' ties to plants

Imagine growing up in a culture in which it was common to hear plants speaking to guide us to collect specific species to heal particular illnesses and medical conditions. Imagine that these direct communications from the plants were honored as coming from sacred beings who communicated their intelligence to us through dreams and visions, and that everyone in the community believed them and honored these forms of subtle interspecies communication.

A wonderful example of this is described by author and teacher John Perkins. Perkins, an economist and management consultant to large corporations and the federal government, was interested in learning about spiritual and ecological practices from a variety of teachers from indigenous cultures, particularly in South America. In one of his stories, Perkins relates how Manco, a master teacher to some of the Quechua shamans, accepted an invitation to visit Perkins and his family in the United States. While visiting, this Ecuadorian shaman provided many healings to close friends of Perkins. Perkins describes how his daughter Jessica introduced Manco to the various plants in their backyard. Manco found some plants that he recognized and many that he had never seen before. "Now," he told Jessica, "You will learn how to talk with the plants when you don't already know them. The first step: You must be them."[3]

After Jessica went to school, the Ecuadorian healer spent the rest of the day "psychonavigating into the different plants." When Perkins asked him how he was able to receive information about the healing and medicinal value of the plants he had never seen before, Manco said, "Just sit here in front of this little flower," pointing at a heavenly blue morning glory. "Let your spirit join its spirit. Merge your energy fields. . . . All you have to do is journey into a plant, be it, and learn its secrets."[4] He told Perkins that the necessary prerequisite was letting go of the "human armor we wear."

We know that our ancestors collectively embraced this nonindustrial epistemology (way of knowing the world), irrespective of their culture or where they lived. That approach is in sharp contrast to the modern approach of Western science, whose primary goals seem to be objectifying and controlling all aspects of the natural world. It is, I think, our enormous loss that we widely regard our predecessors as having been not only unscientific and uneducated, but superstitious and terribly misinformed about the nature of the universe.

As Pollan describes, nutrition science reduces a plant to a handful of useful and "essential" micronutrients that our body needs in order to grow. But the vast majority of nonindustrial cultures had very different ways of gathering information from plants. These methods were based on epistemologies that contained recurrent themes and that were embedded in their cultures. The basic construct of this nonindustrial orientation is made up of a number of overlapping beliefs, including the following[5]:

- What contemporary physicists now believe is essentially what our ancestors were saying—that there is a unifying force that connects all things in the universe. Quantum physicists call this the *quantum field* or *Mind of God,* while ancient peoples frequently called this central platform underlying all things *The Great Spirit.*
- Everything emerges from and is made from this central unifying principle, such that the sacred is manifested in physical matter.
- It naturally follows that since the sacred is in all things, soul or sacred intelligence is in all things as well.
- Since humans are a part of this sacred intelligence that all things share, we have the capacity to use that intelligence to communicate with plants, animals and all other matter.

Similarly, other intelligences or souls have the ability to communicate directly to humans.

- Humans arrived on Earth after other plant and animal organisms, so we have much to learn from these other intelligences. They have new information (or ancient information not yet disseminated) about the natural world to teach us.

- Just as every human being expresses more or less of their inherent sacredness, so too do specific locations throughout Earth. To the degree that we choose to consciously cultivate second attention awareness of or ongoing mindfulness of our environment, we can become more sensitive and receptive to sacred communication from the earth (and other natural intelligences) that are trying to convey important information to us about healing.

- Humans are just a part of the interconnected web of all life on this planet, and all members of this sacred intelligence will benefit from us continuing to acknowledge and honor this truth.

These beliefs summarize the cross-cultural epistemological orientation of nearly all of our ancestors throughout the world, highlighting the underlying theme of the profound interrelationship of humankind with the earth and all things in the universe. Our ancestors did not feel isolated, nor did they suffer from the more modern malaises known as depression and anomie. *For them, the earth truly was magical and all things were alive with Spirit.* Native North Americans were among those who cherished the plant world for the healing knowledge the plant spirits shared with them. The ethnographic research literature shows that this was true in nearly every

> Humans are just a part of the interconnected web of all life on this planet, and all members of this sacred intelligence will benefit from us continuing to acknowledge and honor this truth.

tribal group. The Cherokee and the Creek people, for example, had an intimate relationship with the plant world. It was understood among them that the plants had compassion for their human offspring, "and that each plant offered up a remedy to heal one of the diseases of humankind."[6] Embedded in their cultural epistemology was that plants are our teachers and healers.

These truths were not based on myth. They were based on our ancestors' ability to enter into "non-ordinary states of being" that their survival depended on. Renowned anthropologist Michael Harner has researched and described these different states of consciousness and asserts that they juxtapose our everyday "ordinary reality" orientation. The different states of consciousness that we are not normally accustomed to experiencing or perceiving were accessed by shamans in indigenous cultures via "non-ordinary reality." Ritualized shamanic journeys enabled them to relate directly to the spirits of the plants and animals for information and knowledge pertaining to healing.

Since the early 1980s, when Dr. Harner established the Foundation for Shamanic Studies, thousands of people (including myself) have been trained in this ancient methodology, giving us moderns the same abilities to allow us access to the seemingly magical world of non-ordinary reality. While in this easy-to-access altered state of consciousness, one can immediately perceive and understand that plants are sentient beings that respond to our thoughts and intentions. Scientific researchers have confirmed that plants can respond to shifts and changes in their ecosystem with immediate modifications to their own biochemistry, creating new chemical compounds that are necessary for adaptive survival. To add credence to our ancestors' paradigm,

> when researcher Clyde Baxter connected a lie detector
> to a plant, he was astonished that it could tell from his
> thoughts what his intentions were when he was going to
> burn it or tear its leaf.[7]

Plants and healing

Our ancestors knew and understood that plants have always offered themselves to us as teachers and healers. Regardless of geographic location, indigenous cultures have always used the local native plants and herbs for supporting, strengthening and healing them. Complementary and alternative medicine are now being used increasingly in the United States. The use of traditional Chinese medicine (the history of which goes back at least 5,000 years) is growing in North America, as acupuncture (and even some traditional Chinese herbal treatments) are now being covered by many health insurance companies.

This phenomenon is the counterpart to the pervasive influence of the pharmaceutical industry. Some researchers claim that one out of every three Americans is now on some kind of antidepressant drug. It has been noted that our water tables are becoming increasingly contaminated by the residues of all these synthetic drugs being excreted and flushed down our toilets. As a result, the food we eat has been irrigated with water that is laden with all kinds of drug residue, since synthetic drugs do not tend to break down in the environment. The long-term consequences of contamination to our biosystems by these synthetic drugs are not known. What is known, however, is that over 100,000 people die each year from the side effects of pharmaceutical drugs, and another 2.2 million "suffer side effects so severe that they are permanently disabled or require long hospital stays."[8]

Scientism has become the prevailing industrial and postindustrial medical paradigm for healing, but plants have always continued to play a prominent role. While many of the pharmaceutical drugs prescribed today are derived from compounds synthesized from plants, there remain millions of people throughout the world who use and attest to the healing value of working with plants directly. An extraordinarily effective method that is available to anyone is flower essence therapy, developed by an English homeopathic physician named Dr. Edward Bach. This therapy can make a major contribution to the support we provide to others and to helping us take better care of ourselves as caregivers.

The plants that called out to an English physician

Dr. Bach (1886–1936) received conventional medical training in London. He began his medical career as a pathologist and bacteriologist in the early 1900s, and developed a number of vaccines for treating intestinal bacteria. After reading Samuel Hahnemann's discourse, *Organon of Medicine*, Bach realized that he agreed with the homeopathic practice of giving minute doses of medicine to patients to stimulate their own regenerative healing powers. Hahnemann, a German physician, developed homeopathic medicine over two hundred years ago. It emphasizes treating the whole person rather than just the presenting symptoms of the disease, and to this day homeopathic practitioners consider physical symptoms, mental factors and emotional factors.

Bach eventually modified the delivery system of his vaccines from injection to minute homeopathic oral doses. However, he continued to be pulled toward a more "nature-based" psychospiritual or holistic healing methodology to support his patients. He began to move away from administering deleterious substances and intestinal bacteria to his patients, even though they were introduced in low doses. Following profound inner guidance, he felt convinced that nature offered a better alternative, and that the answers were in the plant kingdom.

In 1930, Dr. Bach left his homeopathic practice in London to walk the countryside of England. He wanted to learn how the essence or energetic pattern of particular plants could support his patients to come back into mental, emotional and spiritual harmony and balance. Bach had a highly sensitive and intuitive nature, as well as a very unusual ability—he could deliberately put himself into temporary extreme states of emotional and physical distress.

He did this while wandering the countryside, to open himself up to the influences and energetic emanations of the nearby flowering plants and trees. As Bach allowed himself to stay afflicted by a particular emotional and/or physical state of disharmony, he found that he was drawn to the particular plant or flower that he perceived experientially (by physical proximity and physical touch) to balance his extreme state of distress.

Bach then collected the plant material and placed it in a glass dish of spring water for up to three days, allowing the rays of the sun to energize and imbue the water with the essence of the plant or flower. The plant material was then removed from the water, but by that time the water contained the vibrational or energetic signature of the particular plant or flower in a highly condensed form. Once Bach had obtained the original essence of the plant, he created a tincture by diluting it and preserving it (usually in brandy). Bach then administered the plant or flower essence remedy to patients orally, a few drops at a time, or the patients self-administered. Over time, Bach catalogued thirty-eight primary flower essence remedies and a combination remedy called Rescue Remedy, which is composed of five specific flower essences that Bach used and recommended for generalized stress and emergency situations.

> Bach's flower essence remedies act as a catalyst to help dissipate and discharge the underlying and often unrecognized emotional causes of the stressors before they generate the chronic complaints and symptoms that can eventually lead to disease.

Bach dedicated the rest of his life to corroborating that his flower essence remedies successfully balanced the mental and emotional disharmony experienced by his patients. By keeping fastidious research notes of his patients' histories, Bach found that his own experiences in the countryside were replicated again and again by his patients. This research became the basis for what we now know as the Bach flower essence remedies.

Unlike synthetic pharmaceutical drugs, which tend to mask and suppress the symptoms of disease, Bach's flower essence remedies act as a catalyst to help dissipate and discharge the underlying and often unrecognized emotional causes of the stressors before they generate the chronic complaints and symptoms that can eventually lead to disease. Though not widely known in the United States, Bach's flower essences have helped millions of people for over seventy years. Today, they are widely distributed and in over sixty-six countries around the world.[9]

Aligning ourselves with the "soul of nature"

Dr. Bach was a pioneer in psychosomatic medicine. He realized in the 1930s that negative mental attitudes create emotional imbalance, which is often responsible for the onset of disease and physical impairment. He understood how devastating the consequences can be to the human body if unbalanced attitudes and emotions go unchecked. Today, there is a growing subspecialty in medicine—called psychoneuroimmunology—that recognizes this relationship.

As discussed above, we are becoming increasingly separated from our connection to nature and, by inference, the multitude of healing and calming benefits that nature offers us. As a result, we are more prone to ongoing stress, which in turn is increasing the incidence of autoimmune disorders (such as lupus, rheumatoid arthritis and fibromyalgia), heart disease, cancer and diabetes, to name a few. While we cannot so easily disengage from the influences of our culture, we can improve our overall health and well-being by allying with our ancestors' heritage through the use of flower essences.

I believe that Bach has something valuable to teach us beyond his contributions to our understanding of the psychosomatic components of disease. He also recognized that optimal health is supported by acknowledging our soul's purpose and living our lives in accordance with that larger personal destiny, which he exemplified by leaving his medical practice in order to research how flowers and plants can affect our health. He wrote extensively about how psychological and physical symptoms of distress are pointers to something being amiss—namely, that many of us are out of synch with living our life purpose and being in integrity with our Higher Self. Bach was the first to admit that his flower essence remedies were not necessarily an immediate cure-all for his patients' physical symptoms. Being a rather progressive holistic physician for his time, Bach recognized the larger relationship between an individual's personal soul and the larger "soul of nature." His flower essence remedies give us another way—beyond our connections to plants for medicine, food and shelter—to connect our own souls deeply with the soul of nature, and thus experience nature's distinctive healing support. The "soul of nature" is Earth's distinctive life force; the more we are able to merge with it, the more we benefit from its nurturing, supportive energy. Dr. Bach believed that "disease is both preventable and curable . . . it is our fears, our cares, our anxieties and suchlike that opened the path to the invasion of illness."[10]

> We can improve our overall health and well-being by allying with our ancestors' heritage through the use of flower essences.

> Bach recognized the larger relationship between an individual's personal soul and the larger "soul of nature." His flower essence remedies give us another way—beyond our connections to plants for medicine, food and shelter—to connect our own souls deeply with the soul of nature, and thus experience nature's distinctive healing support.

You may recall that Louis Pasteur developed the germ theory as the primary mechanism by which disease occurs. Claude Bernard, a French medical scientist who was a contemporary of Pasteur, challenged the assertion that germs or invading microbes are the primary reason for disease. Bernard believed that it is the state of a person's overall well-being or vitality that determines the degree of receptivity or openness to disease. He noted that the germs Pasteur referred to are widespread throughout the general population, and yet certain people contract the disease or circulating virus while other people do not.

Bernard introduced the idea of resistance to disease. Dr. Bach took this idea a step further. He believed that by using the flower essence remedies we would come into a more holistic balance overall, and that emotional balance increases overall vitality and resistance to disease. Through his own fieldwork, Dr. Bach understood what indigenous people have always known—that we can partner with plants as a way to bring order and profound change to the human psyche and body.

It is true that an agrarian lifestyle and deep connection to the living Earth is no longer an everyday reality for most Western people. But we can still carry on that relationship and support the promptings of our own soul by becoming familiar with the extraordinary benefits conferred on us through Dr. Bach's flower essences. I have been using Bach's flower essence remedies since 1981, and continue to support my clients with them with astounding success. Over the years, I have discovered that there are specific Bach flower essences that show up again and again for different clients (many of whom are caregivers themselves) with the same thematic issues. What follows are specific Bach flower essence recommendations interspersed with some brief case histories of my clients to illustrate their effectiveness for caregivers and helpers, as well as the clients they serve.

Flower essences for caregivers and their clients

To begin, I want to identify particular Bach flower essences that are consistently healing for caregivers and helpers. Although readers who are already familiar with the Bach flower remedies may protest that I have left out significant flower essences that they have used and found to be helpful, it is not my intention nor is it within the scope of this chapter to review the benefits of each of the thirty-eight flower essences. Instead, I am highlighting a small group of Bach's remedies that I believe are relevant to most caregivers and helpers suffering from the challenging long-term effects of supporting others or regularly orienting to the needs of others.

Physical exhaustion and emotional depletion are a frequent complaint among high-intensity relaters. As mentioned in an earlier chapter, it is widely recognized that dedicated and compassionate caregivers and helpers have difficulty saying NO, and therefore have difficulty in maintaining appropriate interpersonal boundaries. This tendency to deny one's own needs and ignore one's own well-being while supporting others is widespread throughout the helping professions. As a clinical supervisor to other therapists and counselors, I have seen this to be true as therapists take on too many clients, see particular clients more often than their schedule realistically and healthily allows, and make themselves overly available by fielding phone calls and e-mails way beyond the agreed-upon therapeutic contract. The symptoms of physical and emotional burnout that these therapists and counselors have, often lead to the onset of disease and emotional depletion, showing up as chronic fatigue, depression and adrenal exhaustion. These individuals often ask the seemingly unanswerable question "Why is there no time in my life for proper self-care and rest?"

The Bach flower essence **Centaury** is specifically indicated to help caregivers who are prone to co-dependency, and who are unable to say NO easily or set proper boundaries with their clients. Whether it's dealing with an elderly parent or an aggressive and self-centered client, **Centaury** supports caregivers to be more assertive and stand up appropriately to people who might otherwise exploit their sensitive and good-hearted nature.

Red Chestnut complements **Centaury** by securing stronger interpersonal boundaries for caregivers who tend to become pre-occupied with worry for the health and safety of those who they are helping and caring for. **Red Chestnut** is helpful for "worst case scenario" thinkers and worriers who become obsessed with and overwhelmed by their concern for others.

It is important to note that while therapists and hospice workers may find these flower essences appropriate for supporting their own care and burnout prevention, the same remedies can be suggested for clients dealing with the same problems in their own lives. For instance, a parent of a teenager who is overtly oppositional and defiant can easily surrender her parenting responsibilities as a way to avoid confrontations with her teenager. While being counseled in the office to say NO and establish better boundaries more con-sistently, **Centaury** is the perfect remedy to support this parent as she consciously works on setting limits with her child. For clients who are dealing with an elderly parent or young child with a chronic illness, **Red Chestnut** is a wonderful and appropriate flower essence to mitigate their ongoing anxiety and worry, allowing them to be more present and thus reducing their distracting mental chatter.

Impatiens flower essence supports practitioners and caregivers to be present and hold the space with clients, even when the client's process is judged to be going "too slowly" or "taking too long." Doctors, therapists and other caregivers often feel pressured by time constraints, managed care imperatives and over-scheduling such that a quick-fix mentality becomes a subtly pervasive under-current in their clinical practice. High-intensity relaters often feel stressed because of the demands of external realities or their own habit of trying to solve problems and figure things out quickly for confused clients so they will immediately feel better. **Impatiens** supports practitioners to get out of their head and be present in the relationship with the other, and to listen actively and deeply to identify the needs and concerns of their client. By using **Impa-tiens**, time can become your ally rather than an oppressive nemesis figure. The energy of **Impatiens** helps you to be more present for your clients, and hold space for them without emitting a vibe of impatience or "let's hurry up and move on to the next thing." Clients can then sense your willingness to really be with their process, and to pay greater attention to the nuances of their healing as new information emerges. This dissipates any of your internally created pressure to push forward quickly, allowing you to appropriately remind your clients that the solution will ultimately emerge from within themselves. **Impatiens** also helps you maintain rapport with your clients by creating a more balanced relational field and subtly conveying that your role is one of facilitator rather than simply fixer. This flower essence provides you with a subtle but powerful reminder that ultimately, clients must deal with and resolve their own issues, even as you, the caregiver, remain committed to supporting and helping them on their healing journey. To summarize, **Impatiens** helps caregivers by enabling greater presence, attentiveness and compassion for the people they are serving.

The next two Bach flower essence remedies speak loudly to provide support to the dedicated caregiver. **Elm** helps caregivers who are overwhelmed by the responsibilities they willingly take upon themselves. While every job has its unique expectations and demands, the responsibilities that high-intensity relaters take on can, understandably, wear them down emotionally. While medical staff working in an emergency room, in an oncology clinic or on an evening telephone hotline deal with life-and-death situations daily, a hospice staffer supporting a dying patient and his family knows in advance that he or she will be dealing with the family's intense grief and loss when their loved one dies. Regardless of how qualified or experienced one may be, the feeling of overwhelm can descend on all types of caregivers like a blanket of dense fog, infusing them with a weariness that slowly takes its toll. When your normal coping abilities can no longer stand up to the pressing emotional demands of these kinds of situations, **Elm** can be a balm that soothes and calms. It can provide a temporary stay in the eye of the storm where you can re-evaluate the situation with greater objectivity.

A close cousin in similar situations is **Oak**. This essence is recommended when the workload or stressor has become too much and a person's ability to carry on against great challenge or adversity destabilizes their homeostasis and they are in danger of imminent emotional or physical collapse. While normally strong and committed to getting the job done "no matter what," many high-intensity relaters veil their vulnerability because their self-identity is wrapped up in staying strong and competent as an example for others. While these caregivers have a strong value system to stay the course regardless of the challenges that confront them, **Oak** can provide them with the strength to complete their tasks while at the same time creating an opening to examine their own needs for rest or consider delegating to others. Sometimes these people are called "pushers" or workaholics; they model to the rest of us extraordinary zealousness and seem to possess unending stores of robust energy, relentless in their determination to prove that anything is possible when other people's well-being is at stake. Yet, even professional athletes must have regular down time in order to prevent exhaustion and depletion. **Oak** supports these caregivers by enabling an energetic shift to take place that subtly reminds the person that occasional time off for recreation and vacation is good medicine for the soul.

There are three other Bach flower essences that every caregiver would be wise to consider.

Crab Apple is widely regarded as the "cleanser." It is frequently indicated for people who feel unclean or ashamed of themselves, either because of something they dislike about their outer appearance or (more frequently) something they have experienced that has created a lingering feeling of being contaminated in some way. These self-perceptions ultimately create a compromised self-esteem or a negative self-image.

For example, a client had been working through old sexual abuse with the added stress of living with an alcoholic partner. Because her father was also an alcoholic, the memories and feelings that were brought up associated with her childhood sexual abuse were intensified by being around her current alcoholic partner. This client repeatedly reported feeling dirty and filled with self-loathing, not just during some of her deep therapeutic releasing and cleansing work in my office but also when her partner became inebriated at home. **Crab Apple** was the remedy of choice. When I saw her again three weeks later, she reported that although things had not changed at home, she was no longer being triggered by her partner's alcoholic binges. Also, in a way that was difficult for her to articulate clearly, she no longer felt dirty when remembering the sexual abuse she had endured decades ago.

In another case, a client of mine who was struggling with compulsive over-eating reported that he continued to feel shame and personal disgust when he lost his resolve and over-ate to the point of physical discomfort. When I saw him four weeks later, he reported that his use of **Crab Apple** in the interim had essentially silenced the inner critical voice that was the underlying cause of the personal disgust and shame he had been feeling. Eventually, with continuing use of **Crab Apple** and energetic boundary work, he was able to bring his compulsive over-eating into control.

While feelings of low self-esteem and negative self-image may be reasons that caregivers reach for **Crab Apple**, it is more likely that this remedy will be called for when caregivers feel they have been contaminated by their clients' negative emotional energy. This can be a very subtle process, and I have discovered in my training program (and written about extensively in my first book, *Dynamic Energetic Healing*®)[11] that many therapists have not cultivated the sensitivity or self-awareness to make a direct connection (in their conscious awareness) between what happened during an interaction with a client and their subsequent feeling of being contaminated by psychotoxic emotional energy.

As I detailed in my first book, subtle negative energy is often a consequence of significant trauma that, like a parasite, energetically burrows into a person's biofield and creates persistent problems. These problems can culminate with an array of symptoms, including insomnia, free-floating anxiety, unusual physical symptoms of distress that are difficult to diagnose, and post-traumatic stress disorder. I teach my trainees and the therapists I supervise proper energetic and psycho-emotional hygiene to prevent any type of this contamination from occurring as a consequence of interactions with clients. For example, clients who are extremely agitated and angry, or clients who describe in detail horrific traumas that happened to them (such as physical battering, ritual abuse or rape) create a strong potential for vicarious trauma. They also leave a palpable and persistent feeling in the caregiver or therapist of not being able to separate themselves from the events their clients described, and as a result the caregiver feels dirty or contaminated after the client has left. In these kinds of cases, **Crab Apple** is exactly the right Bach flower essence to help caregivers release and process their experience of being contaminated. Note that **Centaury** and **Red Chestnut** can be used simultaneously with **Crab Apple** to support an individual who is also experiencing compromised boundaries and preoccupation with worry for their client.

When someone is suffering from the effects of shock, trauma or personal loss, **Star of Bethlehem** is indicated as the remedy to help restore emotional balance. While high-intensity relaters must constantly work on maintaining good interpersonal boundaries, no doubt there will still be times when a severe trauma or loss suffered by a client affects the caregiver vicariously. There will also be times when the caregiver herself is going through a major loss or traumatic event that will destabilize her, making it difficult to be fully present for her clients. **Star of Bethlehem** is called for, since the specific pattern from this plant essence provides comfort and restores emotional equanimity.

One of the wonderful consequences of practitioners becoming familiar with and using Bach flower essences is that they can then make appropriate recommendations to clients. For example, a client of mine found that **Star of Bethlehem** helped her enormously in dealing with her grief at the loss of her mother. Another client who lost her father found that because of the dominating and controlling personality he had, she needed both **Star of Bethlehem** and **Centaury** to help her deal with her feelings of loss and what she perceived to be the lingering intrusive demands made by her deceased father's spirit while she struggled to come to terms with their relationship during the weeks following his death.

Bach flower essences and stalking the critic

In Chapter 6, I discussed the importance of "stalking" your inner critic as a way to prevent self-sabotage. In addition to the strategies mentioned there, there are a few flower essence remedies that can help you silence your inner critic.

One of my clients, Camille, was struggling with feelings of overwhelm at the thought of having to consistently confront her inner critic. She had realized that there seemed to be a relationship between her inner critic and her now-deceased, controlling and verbally abusive father. She had been stalking the critic and journaling about her daily progress for a couple of weeks, as well as fanning in front of her solar plexus chakra every day. But I realized that she needed additional support to prevail over this historically powerful condemnatory judge.

I suggested that a Bach flower essence might be appropriate for Camille. I had in mind a few particular essences that might be helpful: **Pine**, for when you feel guilty or are blaming yourself; **Rock Rose**, for feelings of extreme terror about something; **Beech**, for when you feel critical or intolerant toward other people; and **Larch**, for when you expect to fail or lack confidence in yourself.

We muscle tested all thirty-eight primary remedies individually using a blind procedure (neither of us knew which label was on which bottle). The only Bach flower essence that muscle tested strong for Camille was **Larch**. Upon further muscle testing inquiry, it was determined that taking **Larch** twice a day for the next two weeks would support Camille to have solid energetic boundaries with her inner critic, and help her depotentiate the critic as she built up her stores of personal power, confidence and overall vitality.

Emergency relief

The last flower essence that is important to know about is **Rescue Remedy**, which is the only combination of essences formulated by Dr. Bach himself. This combination remedy was carefully developed for those emergency stress situations that demand immediate attention—when there is little or no time to consider which individual flower essence would be best for the given situation. Though none of the flower essences should be considered a cure-all for any situation, **Rescue Remedy** can be taken immediately after hearing bad news or experiencing a significant fright or accident. It can also be taken just before a difficult or challenging situation, such as taking an exam or speaking in front of a crowd. In addition to **Star of Bethlehem** and **Impatiens**, **Rescue Remedy** includes **Cherry Plum** (indicated for when one fears losing control of oneself or acting in an irrationally angry or possibly violent manner), **Rock Rose** (for when one feels terror-stricken, helpless or panicky verging on hysteria), and **Clematis** (for when one dissociates from present reality and becomes spaced out, dreamy and preoccupied with a desire to escape the present situation). I always have a bottle of **Rescue Remedy** on hand at home, and make certain to have it with me whenever I travel, either alone or with my family.

Using Bach's flower essences

Dr. Bach's flower essence remedies are safe, gentle and effective. They can be purchased at most health food stores or directly over the internet. Their manner of application and use couldn't be easier. Sold in three-quarter ounce amber bottles preserved with a small amount of alcohol, the usual dose is four drops in a cup of water four times a day. For those people averse to alcohol, the drops can be put directly on the skin, used as a spray or even put in a bath. As Bach himself asserted,

> As all of these remedies are pure and harmless, there is
> no fear of giving too much or too often, though only
> the smallest quantities are necessary to act as a dose.
> Nor can any remedy do harm should it prove not to be
> the one actually needed for the case. [12]

Remember, it is the vibrational pattern inherent in the plant from which the essence is derived that creates the healing responses. Having worked with the Bach flower essences for nearly thirty years now, it becomes quite apparent to me which essence or essences would be most helpful for my clients at any given time. Since I include behavioral kinesiology as an integral part of my therapy model, I frequently muscle test a client's arm while he or she holds the bottle(s) in their other hand to corroborate for them that the essence I have selected strengthens their system in relationship to their particular issue. I then spend a few minutes helping them to fashion a brief statement of affirmation along with a positive and healing image for them to incorporate while ingesting the Bach flower essence. That helps to seed the client's subconscious mind with a positive statement of intent, accompanied by an image of themselves healed of their particular issue or malady. Thus, this approach recruits their active imagination and engages new thought patterns to accelerate their change process into a new and more constructive reality.

If you do not have access to a practitioner who practices muscle testing, spend some time reading through the guide that accompanies most Bach flower remedies. The guide is usually available at the store where the Bach flower essences are sold, and can also be bought over the internet. The guide lists all the remedies and the specific emotional issues that the particular remedy balances. If you are unsure which remedy is the best one to use, you can select two that both seem to address the issue you need support with. As Bach said, no remedy can cause you any harm if it is not the one that will create the balancing action.

If the issue a client is dealing with requires more support or self-nurturance, I also recommend gently fanning a few inches in front of the heart chakra (for illustrations and discussion of the chakras, see *Dynamic Energetic Healing*®).[13] If the issue they are struggling with is related to interpersonal boundaries and a lack of feeling empowered (see Chapter 7), I suggest that they gently fan a few inches in front of their solar plexus chakra immediately after they ingest the Bach flower essence, while simultaneously affirming and imagining themselves already healed.

Frequently, only one Bach flower essence is recommended at any given time. Yet it is not unusual for two or sometimes three flower essences to be selected and used simultaneously. Dr. Bach stressed that his remedies could be used in combination with any other form of treatment—they complement other approaches rather than interfere with them.

Since I usually see clients every three to four weeks, they use the Bach flower essences as initially recommended for the duration of the time between appointments. The exception to this is when **Rescue Remedy** is used for an emergency stress situation. Because the need for **Rescue Remedy** is usually situational rather than ongoing, the length of time it should be taken depends on the particular stressor.

Dr. Edward Bach was unusual for his time. He was trained as a licensed physician, but his awakened spiritual nature compelled him to turn to the natural world when he was searching for a way to stay connected to his wholeness and respect the whole person.

In response to an inquiry about the preparation required for the flower essence remedies, Bach remarked:

> Let it be noted in this that the four elements are involved: the Earth to nurture the plant; the air from which it feeds; the sun, or fire to enable it to impart its power; and water . . . to be enriched with its beneficent magnetic healing.[14]

As Bach's flower essences have become more widely recognized for their remarkable balancing and healing qualities, other groups of people throughout the world have developed their own compilations of local flower essences, from California to Australia. While every flowering plant has its own special healing qualities, the Bach flower essences remain the original flower essence templates with universally recognized, time-tested efficacy. I invite you, regardless of the healing context in which you provide care or help, to explore and experience flower essences for yourself. You will be amazed and delighted by your new healing allies as you discover an accessible way to reconnect with the natural world here in the twenty-first century. While the Bach flower remedies may at first seem too simple a solution (and thus initially difficult to embrace), you won't find an easier or more effective way to support yourself and maintain your own well-being in your work with caring for others.

Questions and Exercises

1. How do you experience your connection to the natural world? Some people fill their house with plants, others hike or bike on nature paths. Vegetable gardeners revisit the miracle of life annually by tenderly planting seeds in the warming spring soil and happily harvesting the bounty that Mother Earth so graciously provides for our sustenance. What are the ways in which you connect to the natural world?

2. Do you talk to your plants? Do you sense that your house-plants or garden vegetables respond to your thoughts? Do you care about your plants with the same love and concern that you do for your pets (should you be lucky enough to have any)? If not, consider deepening your relationship to your plants by communicating with them often, either mentally or even by talking to them. Notice what changes.

3. While pharmaceutical drugs are widely prescribed by doctors, many people today continue to use natural herbal remedies. Are there any herbal remedies that you like to use? Though you might not think about it too much, one way that many people connect to the natural world is through a soothing cup of tea (which is made using the flowers and leaves of the tea plant). Many people use green and black teas for their caffeinated power boost and to increase their intake of antioxidants, take peppermint tea to aid their digestion, use stinging nettles to manage their allergies, and drink chamomile in the evening to help them relax prior to sleep. Consider trying or adopting a new herbal tea and notice what happens.

4. When you become aware of the intrusive voice of your inner critic, what feelings emerge when you begin to talk back to it? Review my suggestions about using specific Bach flower remedies. Do you think one of them would be helpful in supporting you to speak up and silence that critic? Native peoples throughout the world claim that every plant has its own intelligence or spirit. Consider that there is a particular plant intelligence that can help you become more at peace with your own negative inner chatter.

5. Is there a particular place that you are continually drawn back to because of its unique beauty or sense of nurturing calm? Many people believe that there are some unusually "power

filled" places along the electromagnetic ley lines of Earth, where our planet's life force energy is especially strong and vibrant. On the island of Hawaii where the active volcano Kilauea continues to spill its lava into the ocean, my experience of the life-giving force of Gaia is especially powerful. Whenever I visit the Big Island, a part of me feels that I'm home. Where is it that you feel most connected to the earth?

9

Optimize Your Self-Care by Managing Your Chi

Cultivate chi awareness

In Chapter 7, the concept of chi (the Chinese word meaning *vital force* or *life energy*) was introduced briefly. There, I discussed that having healthy, balanced chi was a necessary component of maintaining healthy energetic boundaries with another person or context. In this chapter, I explore why proper chi management is so important to all aspects of maintaining high level self-care for caregivers, and some steps you can take to strengthen your chi and keep it flowing. Learning about the underlying principles of the traditional Chinese medicine model is an effective way for you to deepen your understanding of how best to work with your chi, which is an important component for taking care of yourself and preserving your health as a high-intensity relater.

Licensed Chinese medical doctors support and augment the body's own healing resources by using a combination of therapies and treatments, including acupuncture and Chinese herbs. They sometimes also recommend exercises for keeping the patient's chi balanced, such as qigong or tai chi quan, as a way to support the acupuncture interventions done in the office. The underlying goals of Chinese medicine are essentially about creating harmony in one's life by gathering, circulating, properly using and conserving our chi. While all of these aspects are implemented and addressed when one visits a doctor practicing traditional Chinese medicine, it is then up to the patient to maintain and strengthen the flow of their chi between visits. This is done by taking the recommended Chinese herbs, establishing and maintaining a proper diet, getting enough rest and, if directed, integrating specific exercises (as mentioned above) that recruit and promote the circulation, purification and conservation of chi for sustaining health.

The primary orientation of Western medicine tends to be treating the symptoms of disease, whereas Chinese medicine has a very different emphasis. It is based on the patient taking greater personal responsibility to enhance his or her own health in order to prevent disease. When you see a practitioner of Chinese medicine to get an initial diagnostic assessment, she will initially look for signs that reflect the current state and condition of your chi. Typically, if your vital force is strong and flowing, you

- feel rested, sleep well, and have good stamina
- feel happy or inwardly peaceful
- have few complaints of pain
- experience that *all* aspects of your life—including your relationships and emotions—are in proper balance

In contrast, if your chi is deficient, stagnant or imbalanced, you probably feel stressed and

- experience tension, insomnia and fatigue
- are troubled with emotional lability, including feelings of anger, depression, anxiety and fear
- have a tendency to be sick frequently with colds and flu
- suffer with degenerative and disabling disease
- are bothered by different experiences of physical pain[1]

Balance and harmony are motifs expressed in many Chinese art forms as well as in Chinese medicine. When your chi is strong and flowing well, you experience harmony within yourself and in relation to your outer world. When you are relaxed, your chi is flowing without restraint, which in turn means that all aspects of your being are nourished. The accumulation of chi can occur spontaneously if your life is not overly stressed. The balance that we all strive for results from maintaining sufficient stores of chi and is usually something that can only happen if we set the intention to establish some kind of daily practice to promote a lifestyle of balance and harmony.

> When your chi is strong and flowing well, you experience harmony within yourself and in relation to your outer world. When you are relaxed, your chi is flowing without restraint, which in turn means that all aspects of your being are nourished.

The fundamental principle on which this book is based is that high-intensity relaters, who tend to be more empathic and sensitive (especially to external stimuli), must deliberately exercise excellent self-care. Since maintaining your body's healthy chi is a crucial aspect of preserving your health and well-being, it is important that you learn to recognize the signs that indicate the current state of your chi, and learn techniques to strengthen and improve the flow of this vital energy.

For example, consider your relationship with the daily media. When you spend time at your computer or in front of a television screen, your energy (that is, your chi) is being recruited to direct your attention to the stimuli coming from the screen. Over time, this depletes your overall energy, since very little positive energy is being exchanged. In fact, the electromagnetic radiation from electronic appliances has been shown to be deleterious to the human energy system.[2] In addition, the extended sedentary activity places physical

> The fundamental principle on which this book is based is that high-intensity relaters, who tend to be more empathic and sensitive (especially to external stimuli), must deliberately exercise excellent self-care.

stress on your body, which further compromises your chi. If sitting at your computer for countless hours causes physical tension in your low back or shoulders and neck, this muscle tension will block the flow of healthy chi circulating throughout your body. This can result in chronic physical complaints and, if ignored for too long, can result in serious back problems or disease.

If at the end of a long workday you choose to watch a movie or some television program, ask yourself: What is the state of my nervous system and my chi? Am I feeling tired, exhausted, energized or restless? Do I, as the guardian of my nervous system, need to take a walk or exercise, lie down and get quiet in a dark room, retreat by reading a novel, or forget about my day by getting lost in a multimedia experience? Will whichever activity I choose risk overstimulating my already stressed sympathetic nervous system and deplete my chi?

If you are someone who would rather, for example, have a glass of wine with dinner and hang out with your family in the evening, ask yourself: What is going on with my body? What does my body feel like it needs?

Your body will not betray you if you stay in relationship with it. Take the time to check in with your body consciously, and learn to interpret the messages it sends you. How your body (and, more specifically, your nervous system) feels reflects the state of your chi. Checking in regularly may sound like a fairly easy thing to do, but many people are quite out of touch with their own body. We all tend to get into routines, and gradually these routines become habits. Once you have formed a habit, your reflective and critical thinking tends to become suppressed, and you begin to ignore or discount the signals your body is giving you about the state of your chi. You ignore these signals at your peril.

> Your body will not betray you if you stay in relationship with it. Take the time to check in with your body consciously, and learn to interpret the messages it sends you.

As a caregiver, it is typical for you to expend much of your store of chi by caring for and supporting others for at least eight hours during the day. Working regularly with demanding, angry or depressed people exposes high-intensity relaters to toxic "energy drainers" (such as the energetic vampires and drama queens discussed in Chapter 7) who spread their psychotoxic energy and drain your chi from you. Being completely present for someone else, hour after hour, can take its toll.

Energetic boundary issues are absolutely related to how you protect (or give up) your chi. If your boundaries are weak, they will not be able to protect you from the psychotoxic energy directed at you by clients who are energy drainers. Their possessive or demanding qualities energetically embed themselves in your physical body and energy field, gradually draining away your chi. This can have dire long-term health consequences if you are not sensitive to the energetic component of your work as a caregiver or helper. Chi depletion is the predecessor of disease—make no mistake about this. Many people who suffer from chronic fatigue or adrenal exhaustion have insufficient boundaries with one or more individuals with whom they regularly interact. In many cases, although these boundary issues are often the primary ongoing cause of their illness, they have never been addressed directly. This is why the primary directive to take care of yourself first is so essential. Embedded in this primary directive is the imperative to protect and conserve your chi. If you do not, you will unwittingly (and regrettably) become cumulatively drained and physically depleted. This occurs because you are not working with your vital force consciously.

Much like becoming conscious of your empathy, becoming conscious of the state of your chi is a necessary part of your self-care. You may feel delighted with yourself and your joie de vivre, and congratulate yourself on being able to give and give of yourself to others. But are you truly conscious of the state of your chi? If not, one day you may well

> Becoming conscious of the state of your chi is a necessary part of your self-care.

discover that just like the unawareness inherent in unconscious empathy and the consequences that emerge from it, you have, in fact, been unaware of the ongoing status of your chi and now must suffer the consequences of allowing your vital energy to become depleted.

General tools for the long-term maintenance of healthy chi

In the Chinese medicine paradigm, the accessibility of your chi is limited only by your awareness and intent. We all tend to become overly focused on our day-to-day routines and responsibilities, which often blinds us to the beauty and miraculous nature of our existence. The chi-enabling Chinese medicine model explains that if we would only take the time to expand our usual narrow focus on our responsibilities to a more all-encompassing awareness, we would discover that nourishing chi is plentiful and widely available. By opening up our awareness to be receptive, we will discover that the natural world is a bountiful provider of sustaining chi. By *redirecting our intent*, we can absorb the life-nourishing chi from the sun, the trees and plants in our yard and parks, the living earth that sustains the plant life on the planet, and the water from the rivers, oceans and rain. By opening up our awareness with appreciation, we can take in the nourishing chi from the fresh fruits and vegetables we grow, select and prepare. This hard-to-measure aspect of our sustainable nutrition is quite different from the phytonutrients that scientists believe plant foods provide to us.

> By opening up our awareness to be receptive, we will discover that the natural world is a bountiful provider of sustaining chi.

And what about the air element? While I recommend the practice of deep breathing for relaxation and reducing stress, consciously breathing in the vital life force that permeates the universe *with intent* is one of easiest and most consistent ways to tap into the endless supplies of chi that is always readily available. When I was regularly practicing and learning Kundalini Yoga, I discovered that a subset of the practice was consciously inhaling and exhaling my breath to charge my nervous system, balance my chakras and provide sustained, balanced mental and emotional energy. This practice is called *pranayama*. The Indian word *prana* has the same meaning as the Chinese word *chi*, which reflects a cross-cultural awareness that this vital force permeates all things and can be accessed and used in intentional ways when we consciously intend to nourish ourselves daily.

Not everyone can find the time to practice qigong, tai chi quan or yoga regularly. Luckily, there are many other practices that can be implemented every day to support the healthy maintenance of your vital energy. What follows are some suggestions for day-to-day habits you can strive to cultivate in order to augment your chi as a powerful way to preserve your health and maintain your well-being.

Stay hydrated

If you're going to be working with and balancing your life energy, you need healthy cells and optimal biochemical reactions in your physical body. In turn, this means that you must be well hydrated. It is estimated that your body is about 70 percent water. Blood is made up mostly of water, and your muscles and organs (such as your lungs and brain) are all composed of significant percentages of water. Your body needs sufficient stores of water to regulate your body temperature and to provide the means for nutrients to travel to all your organs. Water also transports oxygen to your cells, removes waste products, and protects your joints and organs. Alternative healthcare practitioners have long advocated the importance of staying well hydrated, and this truth is becoming more evident within the established medical community as well. "It takes at least six to eight cups of pure water each day to keep the skin and body well hydrated," notes Dr. Jeanette Jacknin, a dermatologist and author of *Smart Medicine for Your Skin*.[3] Many healthcare practitioners believe that there is an epidemic of chronic dehydration. Along with the symptoms of thirst, dry skin, and fatigue, other problems from insufficient hydration can include premature aging and digestive disturbances.[4]

Good hydration in your body also helps to keep your energy system running efficiently. Applied kinesiology practitioners have consistently empirically verified that optimal circulation of chi is enabled and enhanced when clients are well hydrated. So go ahead—have a glass of water and visualize taking in life-giving chi that circulates and distributes itself throughout your body. It is one easy way to continually replenish yourself during the day.

Get enough rest

Integrating regular rest and relaxation into your daily life seems like a reasonable expectation if you want optimal health and well-being. But many of us have such demanding schedules that getting enough rest sometimes seems impossible.

Some people can regularly get by on four to five hours of sleep per night, but researchers continue to discover how essential adequate sleep is for keeping all of our mind-body systems operating optimally.

How much sleep should you get? There is a lot of conflicting research about how many hours per night is best. If you feel sufficiently energized to accomplish everything that your busy day requires of you, you are probably getting enough sleep. On the other hand, if you find yourself regularly complaining about being tired, the first thing to consider is modifying your schedule so that you get more sleep, even if it means eliminating some of your routinized evening activities despite all the temptations to retain them. Sleep deprivation can lead to a host of problems, including increased need for caffeine to chemically compensate for chronic tiredness and the disruption of essential hormones that regulate blood sugar, appetite and mood.

Statistics continue to reveal that the stresses of the twenty-first century are good business for the pharmaceutical companies that manufacture and sell sleeping pills.

> A recent review of prescription drug claims of 2.4 million Americans between 2000 and 2004 by Medco Health Solutions, a prescription drug benefit management company, found that among adults aged 20 to 44, use of sleep medications doubled while the use of sleeping pills among children aged 10 to 19 jumped 223 percent. All told, Americans filled 35 million prescriptions for sleeping pills in 2004 at a cost of $2.1 billion.[5]

Note that the above quote refers to data collected before the economic meltdown of 2008. As I write this at the end of 2011, it is likely that now even more people are experiencing financial and employment worries that affect their sleep.

In fact, one of the most daunting problems I encounter in my private practice is trying to help clients who complain about sleep issues and want to find out what is causing them. While there are often specific trauma-related reasons that generate the anxiety and worry that keep people awake at night, lifestyle choices and overwork are usually primarily responsible for poor sleeping patterns. With all the responsibilities people have to confront at work and at home, there often is little time to wind down and truly relax after dinner is prepared and the kids are in bed. This is particularly true for high-intensity relaters, who absolutely need to create a healthy end-of-the day routine for self-care and calm.

There are various ways to increase your likelihood of getting enough rest. Consider the following suggestions for making this happen for yourself.

- The most obvious first step is to acknowledge that you feel better throughout the day when you are getting sufficient sleep. This acknowledgment in itself creates the incentive to make a plan.

- Commit to making it a priority to maintain a regular bedtime.
- Get enough physical activity or exercise during the day. Sitting at a desk can become very tiring after many hours, but it doesn't count as exercise! Your body needs to move, whether just by walking or by following a regime at the gym. Monitor how late you can tolerate vigorous exercise without it making you so overstimulated that it interferes with your ability to fall asleep. I exercise at the gym regularly, but have discovered that if I work out after 5 PM I am too amped up for the rest of the evening and have a hard time falling asleep at my normal bedtime.
- Try taking a short nap during the day. Every day at around 4 PM, my biorhythms inform me that I must rest and reset my biocomputer for a short time. I become sleepy and find it difficult to concentrate. Thanks to my many years of practicing yoga, I can lie down, close my eyes and immediately go into a deep state of relaxation that is a dream-like trance state. Although I am not actually asleep, I am aware of my mind and thoughts unwinding and processing many of the issues I have been working on and thinking about during the day. Within minutes, I can feel my body sinking into the floor, completely letting go of all my accumulated physical stress. I rarely need more than fifteen or twenty minutes, and when I am done I truly feel rejuvenated. I have clear and sustained mental energy until late in the evening. If you do not already do this, give yourself permission to try it. You will likely be pleasantly surprised.
- Establishing a bedtime routine sends a message to your body that you are preparing or priming it for sleep. As a high-intensity relater, this fits in well with your temperament. Move away from the computer or bright television screen

and make a point of reducing the light level around you. This tells the ancient part in your brain that your workday is nearing its end and the sun has gone down. Sleep scientists know that bright lights can suppress levels of the hormone melatonin, making it harder to fall asleep. Perhaps a hot bath, quiet meditation or even reading a book under a small book lamp will work. Take care of any unfinished emotional business with your partner so you are calm, resolved and ready to let go of the business of the day. These actions help to calm your nervous system and signal both your mind and your body that you are now ready for sleep.

- If you feel you just can't unwind, consider over-the-counter herbal supplements such as melatonin and valerian. There are numerous nonpharmaceutical alternatives that your naturopath or pharmacist might recommend. Everyone's situation and body chemistry are different, so do your own research and consult a healthcare professional whom you trust. He or she can provide the proper guidance and monitoring to help you achieve regular, restful sleep.

Once you are getting enough rest on a regular basis, you will be providing your physical body with the opportunity to build up its stores of chi, enabling you to be the very best you can be physically.

Eat fresh, healthy foods

Purchasing and consuming fresh and healthy foods that are devoid of toxic chemicals is certainly part of a disciplined daily health regimen that will support you and help you gather excellent vital life force. Fresh plants are full of chi from the earth, which they emanate and make freely available to us. The more you appreciate their freshness, beauty and vitality consciously (rather than just

> Fresh plants are full of chi from the earth, which they emanate and make freely available to us.

commenting on how expensive they are), the more you create an energetic bond between yourself and that source of food. You might even take a moment to mentally thank the plant for absorbing the energy of the sun, water and air and then providing it to you, thus enabling you to directly and immediately benefit from taking in this vital energy. As I stated in an earlier chapter, preparing fresh and healthy food is a celebration of the miraculous nature of our connection to the earth. The more gratitude and appreciation we feel, the greater is the benefit and penetration of chi that we ingest from food.

Shopping for and preparing organic fruits and vegetables is just as much a discipline as a daily qigong or tai chi quan practice. It is a regular reaffirmation of your intention to care for yourself after spending so much time during your workday caring for others. Spend a little more money to buy high quality food. You're worth it!

Ask a holistic health practitioner to recommend herbs and natural supplements

It is beyond the scope of this book to recommend specific herbs and supplements (other than valerian and melatonin for sleep), since the choice of supplement and the quantity of it that you take are determined based on your unique body and circumstances. However, I can make the general statement that using health-promoting herbs and supplements supervised by a holistic health practitioner is another significant way to augment your chi.

If you can afford it, consider working with a naturopath or practitioner of Chinese medicine. Their orientation may be a better fit for you than that of a doctor of Western medicine, since naturopaths and Chinese medicine practitioners are trained to support your physical body nutritionally with herbs, diet and supplements.

By working regularly with a well-qualified person you trust, you can augment any deficiencies that blood tests and persistent physical symptoms may reveal with herbs, food and supplements. Pursuing this as a regular part of your life is a powerful and self-affirming way to support your body and help you avoid potential disease processes that result from untended stress.

Spend time with nature regularly

The Chinese sages have always said that another way to collect and absorb chi is through exposure to the natural elements. When you walk or hike in beautiful natural surroundings, for example, you absorb life-enhancing vital force from the earth, the trees, the running waters of streams and rivers and the infrared warming rays of the sun that penetrate deep into the skin. Caregivers as well as many other working people don't often make time *on a regular basis* to avail themselves of natural, beautiful outdoor environments. But I have found that simply spending time in my backyard garden, pruning my fruit trees, planting seeds and flowers in the earth, or even just sitting under our canopy of oak and fir trees is a wonderful reconnection to the natural world— it is always nurturing for me.

> Caregivers as well as many other working people don't often make time *on a regular basis* to avail themselves of natural, beautiful outdoor environments.

Commit to a daily energetic practice

There are many energetic practices that, when done on a regular basis, nourish the caregiver every day. These practices significantly reduce the risk of falling into the black hole of chronic fatigue or physical depletion. Because I practice qigong and am thus familiar with it, I will use it as my example of one of these energetic practices. The daily practice of qigong involves gentle physical movements accompanied by controlled breathing and specific visualizations. The movements, breathing and visualizations are all designed to stimulate specific acupoints along your energetic meridian system and ensure the free-flowing movement of your chi.

Even today in China, there are hospitals where patients come solely to practice qigong and benefit from traditional Chinese herbs and diet. Patients who are initially too weak to practice the qigong simply lie down next to a group of practitioners so their generation of increased flowing chi will energetically spill over into and permeate those who are too weak to participate actively.

In my first book,[6] I wrote about my first qigong teacher, Master Chen. She began practicing qigong daily when she was no longer able to tolerate the chemotherapy treatment she was receiving for an aggressive form of breast cancer. Master Chen attributes her recovery to this daily qigong practice. It is worth noting that she had never done an energetic healing practice before. But why should you wait until you are struck down by something as terrible as cancer or some other disease? Being proactive is always best.

Qigong is a great practice, but classes in other energetic practices, including tai chi quan and different schools and styles of yoga are also widely available. Consider trying some of these energetic practices until you find the one that feels right for you. The benefits to your overall energy and mood will typically be immediately apparent. Developing the habit of taking time for a daily energetic practice is yet another way to preserve your health and maintain well-being.

> Developing the habit of taking time for a daily energetic practice is yet another way to preserve your health and maintain well-being.

Do less, just "be"

There is another element of the traditional Chinese orientation to being in the world, which has much to do with aesthetics, that is worthwhile mentioning as a way to replenish yourself on an ongoing basis.

The phrases "go with the flow" and "chill out" have become popular slogans that are often associated with certain types of people. For many, these terms apply to individuals who are not necessarily interested in personal achievement or in contributing to changing the world, but instead propound a lifestyle based on never getting riled up or upset. While we can be judgmental toward those who adhere to these ideas, the link between healthy longevity and spiritual inner calm has a long history in Chinese poetry and art.

In those media, this idea is often expressed by the movement of nature juxtaposed with humans, who frequently appear small and insignificant. This is especially evident in landscapes and depictions of moving water in a state of unrestrained flow. These nature-based artistic expressions elicit feelings of balance and harmony where there is no resistance and the beauty or movement of nature predominate. These are implicit teachings, encouraging us to be flexible and accepting of what is happening in the moment, using nature as the metaphoric backdrop. The mythical author Lao Tzu beautifully describes and espouses these themes in his small book of Chinese poetry, *The Tao Teh Ching*. A core tenet of Taoism is the phrase wu wei, the literal meaning of which is "without action," "without effort," or "without control." Wu wei is often mentioned in the context of the paradox *wei wu wei*, which means "action without action" or "effortless doing."[7]

The concept of *effortless action* attempts to describe the paradoxical way of being in the world in which one does not resist or struggle. The goal of this orientation is to experience greater connection with what is happening in the here and now. The idea is that this prevents the constriction or blockage of your flow of chi (which occurs through effort and stress) as you interact with other people and the world. The emphasis is on *being* in the midst of *doing*. This philosophy is in direct contrast to our efforts to try to willfully control or push the process of life in spite of resistance or negative feedback from another person.

Though it may seem paradoxical to most Westerners, inherent in this traditional Chinese orientation to life is the challenge to stay relaxed, do less and *just be*, so that we naturally accomplish more without even really "trying." Part of "accomplishing more" is getting done what you need to without ending up stressed out from over-trying, which requires more reparative therapy after the fact. You may believe that this type of thinking belonged in more innocent and romanticized times in centuries past and is not a viable approach in our fast-paced technological society. But it *is* pressingly relevant and practically applicable for today's caregivers and helpers. It serves as a useful reminder that while answering the call of those who need our help, we should acknowledge that we, too, are part of nature and can work toward being less controlling of the people and contexts we interact with. Of course, this is all about cultivating a different kind of attitude that can become your own inner guiding star throughout your day. How calm can you remain amid all the urgent demands on your time and energy? How willing are you to entertain the possibility that this is achievable and that you can change your life for the better by adopting this attitude?

Andrianna

Andrianna, who has been a hospice nurse for twelve years, was previously a surgical nurse. During that phase of her career, she often felt tired at the end of a long day, but she tended to recover quickly. She knew her role, and she was proud of her knowledge and the acknowledgment she received from the doctors and the surgical staff. She never felt threatened by the demands of her work and liked the challenge.

One day Tony, a good friend of Andrianna's, became ill with can-cer, and Andrianna took on the role of being his medical advocate. She went with Tony to appointments with the surgeon and, eventually, the oncologist. Andrianna knew the territory and felt happy to be there for Tony, who was scared and vulnerable. During this time, she discovered that she liked the deep personal engagement with Tony, who was a patient in need as well as her friend.

Eventually, Tony ended up in the hospice ward. Andrianna had never been there before—it was a whole new world for her. At first she was a bit wary and even overwhelmed. But because of her love and caring for Tony, she discovered that her presence had a calming effect on him.

Andrianna also came to realize that she had the same calming effect on a number of other patients. She began to make herself available for fielding questions and helping them to navigate through this scary and unfamiliar medical terrain. Gradually, Andrianna realized that her strong spiritual nature and sensitivity would be well served with patients who were dying.

When Tony finally died, Andrianna had to take a leave of absence from work. She couldn't put her finger on the source of her exhaustion, but just knew she needed a break. She suspected it was an acute grief response, so she started seeing a grief therapist. The therapist helped her to recognize that she was unconsciously over-empathizing with not only Tony but everyone she came into contact with in the hospice ward. Over the course of her therapy, Andrianna came to realize that she needed to make some adjustments in how she related to people, especially in establishing better boundaries. She acknowledged that she was a highly sensitive person, an aspect of her self that had been masked during her years on the surgical ward. Andrianna realized that she had more to offer to people on a one-to-one basis than assisting a surgeon working on an anesthetized patient. She began reading and exploring different approaches to working with the dying.

Andrianna's experience with Tony and the new insight she gained into herself through the grief therapy led her to transfer from the surgical ward to the hospice ward. She quickly discovered that her new job was a busy one that included many different roles and responsibilities. She is always busy meeting new patients, tending to their physical needs and making sure they get the right medications on the right schedule. She also supports their family members, who often don't know what to say to their loved ones and frequently become intensely emotional. When a patient dies, Andrianna counsels the bereaved family members and discusses what preparations are necessary for their loved one's burial or cremation. Clearly, Andrianna meets all the criteria of a high-intensity relater.

When Andrianna started working in the hospice ward, her boundaries were very permeable, although she did not realize it at the time. She came home exhausted and was often affected by secondary traumatization from the extreme grieving of family members, which she had never been exposed to before.

As Andrianna settled into her new job as a hospice nurse, she began going to Vipassana meditation weekend retreats. Soon, she was doing this meditation every night at home. This practice helped her to realize that her primary role was to serve and assist the process of each patient, which she could do best only if she could leave her presumptions and judgments at home each morning. It gradually dawned on her that working with patients who were letting go of the attachments of life meant there was nothing she could do to control their destiny. All she could do was defer to what they needed and help them to be as comfortable as possible. Andrianna realized that since their dying process could not be circumvented, *she* had to let go of her strong desire to direct and control everything that was happening to them. In fact, she came to appreciate that her highest priority was to support her patients to let go of all of their attachments, even to life itself.

> Her primary role was to serve and assist the process of each patient, which she could do best only if she could leave her presumptions and judgments at home each morning.

This new way of thinking was an enormous mental adjustment for Andrianna. It went against all of her training as a surgical nurse, which had emphasized doing everything possible to preserve life. But as a hospice nurse, she gradually became aware that in those cases where she pushed too hard to advocate for a certain intervention, she frequently ran into patient resistance that she simply could not overcome. Though she would not have put it in traditional Chinese medicine terms, Andrianna had discovered how to support her dying patients while surrendering to *their* process as a way to avoid burning out and carrying home resentment.

Over time, Andrianna discovered on her own what *The Tao Teh Ching* teaches about "effortless doing." She couldn't change the various demanding duties and expectations of her job, but she could change her attitude about the job. She gradually adopted an attitude of letting go of control and internally "doing less," which helped her to stay in better ongoing rapport with her patients and their families. She intuitively discovered that her strength as a high-intensity relater was to not always be "doing." Instead, it was to be more present and hold the space for her patients and their families, often taking cues from them for what action was to follow. This discovery came through her native sensitivity and high interpersonal intelligence. No one told her how best to support her patients. She realized that her patients had to determine when they would ultimately let go—it was not up to her.

After two and a half months working as a hospice nurse, Andrianna discovered her energy returning and her previous exhaustion dissipating. She knew she had recovered because she felt different inside—she now felt that she was in exactly the right place where she could be most effective and helpful. She felt that she had discovered something important about the value of human relationships.[8] While she would be hesitant to say this to anyone, she actually felt happy to be with people who were dying because she recognized she had particular gifts that she was using to help these patients prepare for a peaceful transition to whatever was next. She learned to observe herself interacting with her patients and their families through her mindfulness meditation practice and exemplified working without feeling resistance when with her clients by not forcing or judging. She learned how to keep her chi flowing by staying relaxed and maintaining rapport with patients and families. In turn, this approach helped Andrianna to maintain her own health, because she was no longer resisting the flow of life. She also learned how to orient from her heart field through her meditation studies, and literally transformed not just her own life but the lives of many others as well.

I believe that everyone has their own journey to make, and Andrianna's experience reflects what is possible for personal healing and transformation. Her journey toward doing less and "just being" was triggered by her helping her friend Tony, which led her to the grief counseling process. She became aware of how much she enjoyed the deep relating, and developed an understanding of boundaries, grief and the need to not control. Being a classic high-intensity relater, Andrianna then gravitated to work that immersed her in relating deeply to others. She was able to assume her new role easily, not just because deep relating is gratifying but because she was a natural in that role and was drawn to it. Of course, being a hospice nurse is not without its hazards, and Andrianna had many challenges before she came to her self-realization about being more present without controlling and "doing less." The Vipassana meditation helped her to be more centered, learn to hold space for people and not control, and learn to orient from her heart. Going inside, getting quiet and being more present all contributed to her transformation, and she is now living her soul's purpose by serving others from a place of deep compassion. A wonderful consequence of honoring her self while doing her "right work" is that she is not only satisfied on the soul or deep emotional level, but her physical health and overall energy are the best they have ever been.

Eliminate old habits

As qigong master Roger Jahnke has said, "Most interruptions in Qi [chi] circulation that cause disease, discomfort, or dysfunction arise from behaviors, habits, accidents and traumas in life."[9] While it might be argued that we cannot prevent accidents and traumas from occurring in our lives, we can certainly take charge of our behaviors and habits by being more intentional and clear about what we choose for ourselves and our lives. Habits are not always so easy to modify, but so many of my clients, after having cleared and released old traumatic residue, find themselves "suddenly" able to eliminate old, persistent and self-destructive habits and consider establishing new ones. These include stopping smoking and reducing the nightly ritual of over-indulging in alcohol, starting to exercise to reduce physical stress, and initiating healthy dietary regimens after years of habitually eating junk food. Confronting dysfunctional and self-destructive behaviors is always challenging, but choosing to renew a prescription for Xanax (an addictive anti-anxiety drug) is only a short-term solution. This is in contrast to consciously and judiciously examining and ultimately changing the lifestyle that is creating and perpetuating your insomnia, anxiety, chronic headaches and/or other anxiety-related symptoms. Ongoing self-care is really a long-term investment in a lifestyle based on harmony and balance. This requires a willingness to change what we have become habituated to, including our lifestyle.

> Part of the legacy from our ancestors is the accumulated knowledge of how we can consciously and deliberately replenish ourselves daily.

Being aware that what you think and do directly affects how the flow or constriction of your vital life force impacts your health and well-being is another way to conceptualize how important it is for caregivers and helpers to focus on and maintain excellent self-care. Before technology became a part of our lives, people everywhere had to rely on their internal perceptions for practices that would prolong their lives and help to maintain well-being. Over thousands of years of trial and error, people worldwide discovered that living in harmony with the earth provided profound benefits.

I don't want to romanticize the past, given that life without our current technology was hard and often short. But part of the legacy from our ancestors is the accumulated knowledge of how we can consciously and deliberately replenish ourselves daily. To take yoga classes or meditate in the evenings is not just something to brag about over coffee with friends. These and other practical and concrete methods for optimizing chi management are powerful and effective. I have done them in the past and continue to practice them. I have become sensitive to energy or chi over the years from my regular practice of many of these techniques. They are not hard to do and they are available to everyone. Spending more time with the natural world and eating freshly farmed, chemical-free food are things you can do easily if you believe these practices are important—not just for managing or reducing your stress, but to support your essential life force energy, which miraculously keeps your heart beating day after day until the time comes for your body to stop.

Technology is helping us all to live longer, but that does not necessarily mean live better. If the fountain of youth is anywhere, it is all around us in the world, which is permeated by this mysterious and wonderful vital life force, chi. High-intensity relaters have certain predispositions that make them more prone to be open to unhealthy energies or influences that come with relationships. These practices and suggestions are designed to support you to stay strong and empowered. Imagine the possibilities.

Questions and Exercises

1. Traditional Chinese medicine emphasizes managing our vital force or chi as a way to maintain good stamina, overall well-being and longevity. What do you do in your day-to-day life that fosters daily balance and wellness? For instance, do you have a healthcare professional who you consult with regularly to help you create a program for regular exercise, spiritual or energetic practice, or a particular dietary regimen?

2. Are you protective of your vital energy? Are you able to discipline yourself in specific areas of your life in order to nurture and sustain your vital energy? With all the choices of plentiful food and engaging multimedia, do you often find yourself succumbing to seductions that lead you astray from a more conscious and self-determined self-care program? Do you tell yourself that you're just too tired at the end of the day to do anything but eat and collapse on the sofa? Consider integrating one new regular self-care practice to your evenings as a way to cherish and support your vital energy. Post notes around your living space that remind you to implement this practice until it becomes part of your evening routine.

3. Try this new way of thinking about your life: your body is a magical vehicle that is pulsating with the energy and intelligence of the universe. This vehicle can be constantly upgraded and refined, even as you age. If this image resonates with you, try using it as a type of reflective meditation. As part of your regular self-care practice, imagine that the powerful vehicle that is you is continually being refined and perfected. As you breathe in and out, imagine that universal chi is cleansing and refreshing not only every organ of your magical vehicle, but every cell as well. Feel the glow.

4. Have you ever experienced acupuncture or had anyone massage the soles of your feet? The circulation of chi is believed to be just as important as that of our blood. Consider massaging the palms of your hands or the soles of your feet and notice how you feel afterward. Try it with a friend or partner as a way to open yourself to receive from another.

CHAPTER

10

Use Energy Psychology Techniques for Emergency Self-Care

In over thirty years of learning about and working with various psychotherapeutic models, I have found that energy psychology applications are the most consistently effective and efficient interventions for helping clients to create rapid and often immediate changes. This chapter provides a brief overview of energy psychology and how it works, and then focuses on some specific energy psychology *power tools* to augment your self-care repertoire.

The roots of energy psychology are grounded in traditional Chinese acupuncture, which is one of the oldest healing systems that accesses and directs the subtle bioenergy coursing through the human body. Energy psychology has often been called "acupuncture without needles" because the underlying operational principle is based on ancient Chinese medicine methods that relate to accessing chi (see Chapter 9).

Through empirical research over many centuries, the Chinese have precisely mapped out the circulating energy system that's always communicating bioenergetic information throughout the human body. They determined that this energy system includes twelve major meridians or energy channels, each of which passes through a specific organ, such as the kidneys, heart or spleen. Some researchers have proposed that these energy meridians are actually electrical conductors that relay information to and from the brain and the organs via the central nervous system. Acupuncturists primarily use needles on specific acupoints along the twelve major meridians to either stimulate or sedate the movement of chi within and between the meridians, thereby addressing a particular organ imbalance or physiological problem.

The ancient Chinese realized that in addition to coursing through specific muscle groups, each meridian has an emotional correlate. For example, in traditional Chinese medicine the lung meridian is related to sadness and grief, while the gallbladder meridian is related to resentment and rage. As the acupuncturist treats the lungs on the physiological level, the emotion of grief is indirectly being addressed as well.

Detroit chiropractor George Goodheart, who founded the field of applied kinesiology in the early 1960s, studied *Meridians of Acupuncture*, written by British medical researcher Felix Mann in 1964. As Goodheart experimented with adjusting the flow of bioenergy in the body via the classical Chinese meridian system, he discovered that he could balance and strengthen the musculoskeletal system by applying pressure on and tapping various acupuncture points rather than inserting needles.

Soon others were also conducting research in this area, and the evolving field became known as energy psychology (sometimes called meridian therapies). They found that this "needleless acupuncture" was remarkably effective in treating and eliminating negative emotional states and other psychological problems that were caused by the persistent residue of old traumatic experiences and ongoing stress. Foremost among energy psychology's primary researchers were psychiatrist John Diamond, who developed behavioral kinesiology in the 1970s, and psychologist Roger Callahan, who developed Thought Field Therapy® in the mid-1980s. Today, thousands of practitioners around the world participate in international conferences, and new books on the topic are being published regularly.

"Needleless acupuncture" is remarkably effective in treating and eliminating negative emotional states and other psychological problems.

Energy psychology approaches help high-intensity relaters

As I stated in my previous book, "the long-term consequences of trauma frequently emerge as the primary feature from which all subsequent disturbance patterns arise. The tentacles of trauma reach into all areas of people's lives."[1] It has been my clinical experience that when clients request help for anxiety, panic attacks, insomnia or depressed mood, almost always the underlying reason for the genesis of their symptoms is an unidentified trauma. Because trauma is such a familiar part of our lives, many people tend to minimize the persistent and long-term impact of traumatic events, such as a household burglary, an auto accident, a rejection leading to the dissolution of a long-term relationship, or growing up with an alcoholic parent.

Talk therapy, which provides insight into and understanding of why people respond to traumatic experiences like these in predictable ways, is often helpful. However, in many cases it is insufficient for dealing with some of the more complex and intractable consequences of trauma. These include out-of-body dissociation (the situation in which the part of us that carries valuable information about or the memory of a frightening aspect of the trauma is inaccessible to the conscious part of the person's mind); the inability to access certain emotions (frequently known as repression), which creates emotional numbness; and flashbacks and nightmares. People who somaticize repressed feeling states sometimes experience chronic physical symptoms such as migraine headaches, adrenal fatigue, gastrointestinal problems, and other, often crippling physical symptoms attributed to ongoing stress.

Energy psychology theory postulates that psychological problems and persistent traumatic residue reflect disturbed bioenergetic patterns. Energy psychology methods have been developed to help individuals learn to use easily accessible tools to directly and quickly shift these patterns. In energy psychology parlance, when an overwhelming life experience or a traumatic event occurs, a person's energy system becomes disrupted. When this happens, a chi imbalance is created, resulting in symptoms of distress. One way to understand this is that when your essential energy system is flowing freely and unimpeded throughout your body, each of your major meridians is circulating the same amount of energy—in other words, your chi is balanced. When a traumatic event occurs, your bioenergy system may be affected to such a degree that some of the energy in one or more specific meridians becomes depleted or over-energized. This creates an imbalance in the whole interconnected chi matrix.

> In energy psychology parlance, when an overwhelming life experience or a traumatic event occurs, a person's energy system becomes disrupted.

For example, if your energy system is disrupted by your having to stay in a caretaking situation that has become overwhelming, the ongoing imbalance in your energy system will leave you vulnerable and eventually create stress symptoms. Since every situation you encounter throughout your life is encoded and embedded in your nervous system, your body will always remember the event even if your conscious mind does not. If a situation is extremely stressful or traumatic, that information will be stored like a resident file in a computer operating system. This resident file will be running its own mind-body altering program under the radar of your conscious awareness. This under-the-radar storage of trauma-based information in your nervous system always creates an imbalance in your bioenergy system. In some cases, you are aware of these damaging changes right away, while in others you only become aware of the subtle changes after they have had time to accumulate.

It's bad enough that this energy imbalance will perpetuate the symptoms relating to the original traumatic event, keeping you in a state of low-level anxiety or depression indefinitely. What's worse is when a high-intensity relater experiences a new stressful or traumatic event that is similar enough to the original event that it further depletes the energy in one or more of the meridians that were initially affected, which occurs when the *reaction* to the new threat (fight, flight or freeze) is similar to that of the original event. When this happens, it's as though the underlying file (of the original trauma) is now being constantly double-clicked and restimulated, opening up a Pandora's box of multilayered emotional and physical distress that eventually becomes habituated and chronic. This can become an ongoing disruptive influence in your life, and even lead to post-traumatic stress disorder.

Carolyn

For example, consider the plight of Carolyn, a marriage and family counselor. A number of months ago, she had an initial counseling session with a woman whose alcoholic spouse was sometimes threatening. The wife complained about her husband's behavior in the evenings after work, when he habitually drank to the point of getting drunk. When drunk, the husband became loud and belligerent, sometimes threatening her with physical violence if she didn't submit to him sexually. He was unable to discuss anything in a rational manner, and the wife felt desperate and unsafe. When Carolyn heard the woman's story, she recommended that the woman bring her husband to the next session, to try to work things out with some conjoint marital counseling.

During their first session as a couple, the husband immediately began speaking sarcastically to Carolyn, accusing her of conspiring with his wife. As Carolyn tried to redirect the husband's blaming and escalating ranting, she felt her shoulders getting tight, and had fear-induced feelings in her stomach. She managed to keep her cool demeanor and was able to successfully facilitate the couple's dialogue throughout the session. By the end of the session, Carolyn acknowledged to herself that progress had been made—the husband was now aware that his wife was willing to take some serious action to redefine the relationship and stop the abuse. However, Carolyn felt shaken when they left the office.

Carolyn had been in this situation before with angry spouses and had years of experience mediating marital conflicts. Even so, she was shaken up by the overt hostility and loud sarcasm directed at her by the husband. After a few hours, the tension in her body began to dissipate, but she was aware of feeling apprehensive about encountering the couple for another session.

When they came in ten days later, the husband was initially apologetic and contrite. He acknowledged that he and his wife had marital problems and admitted that his drinking had contributed. But when pressed by Carolyn about what he was doing about his drinking problem, he immediately became defensive. The wife interjected that he was still drinking every night, and that she wanted a commitment from him to seek treatment.

The husband became belligerent, and started yelling loudly about how Carolyn was ruining his marriage and he was not going to tolerate it any longer. He got up off his chair and pointed his finger just inches from Carolyn's face, calling her degrading names and getting into a rage. At this point, both Carolyn and the wife stood up and told him to calm down and stop yelling. The husband wheeled around at his wife, screamed "You stupid bitch!" and stormed out of the office, slamming the door behind him. After Carolyn and the man's wife collected themselves, Carolyn recommended that the wife make an appointment to see her alone within the week and discussed what she needed to do to ensure her safety before returning home.

In spite of Carolyn's seasoned experience working with acrimonious couples, she became aware that immediately after the session her breathing was rapid and her chest felt tight. She had a pounding headache and she realized that she was in shock. Carolyn knew from experience that this would probably turn into a migraine headache that could last for forty-eight hours. However, because Carolyn knew how to use energy psychology techniques, she was able to work on herself and come back to emotional homeostasis over a period of a couple of hours.

Immediately following her first encounter with the husband, Carolyn felt shaken up and apprehensive about seeing him again. This first threat had disturbed her energy system and created an imbalance that affected one or more of her acupuncture meridians. In the energy psychology model, when the flow of chi of one or more of the meridians becomes out of balance, the person experiences one or more significant emotional or somatic symptoms that reflect the imbalance. In Carolyn's case, she felt temporary, low-level anxiety that went away by itself after a couple of hours.

During the second counseling session, Carolyn was exposed to the same threat, which that time was even more intense. The initial "file" was double-clicked, and her emotional and somatic reactions were even worse.

In Carolyn's case, it was fortunate that she knew energy psychology techniques that helped her to bring her bioenergy system back into balance. Had she not known how to rebalance her chi using energy psychology methods, the residual shock and negative emotional charge in Carolyn's bioenergy system related to interactions with this man could have become a "resident file," which would be left just waiting to be restimulated. Carolyn's experience with this increasingly hostile and threatening client reflects what can happen to any of us when exposed to a stressor that builds in intensity over time. Often, each subsequent similar interaction (either with this man or with another hostile client who exhibits similar threatening behavior) double-clicks the resident file more quickly, and the symptomatic reactions that occur gradually become more intense. If an underlying "resident file" is left unattended, it could easily become something out of the person's ability to control, and eventually result in post-traumatic stress disorder (PTSD), a most frustrating, persistent and serious condition.

A single traumatic incident is obviously much easier to resolve than numerous similar, interconnected stressors. As the above example with Carolyn illustrates, her first encounter with the angry husband generated stress symptoms that dissipated on their own in just a couple of hours. But when she was threatened more intensely in the second session, this stressor became compounded and her stress symptoms were worse, requiring more attention in order to be resolved. However, energy psychology methods are consistently effective for ongoing events, such as the complex relationship issues that caregivers are most often involved in. Problems that energy psychology applications successfully treat include trauma-related issues such as anxiety and panic attacks, phobias, depression and dissociation, and a host of other emotional and psychological concerns that tend to relate to difficult and often complex relationship issues, such as interpersonal boundaries. Additionally, a host of stress-related physical problems are frequently ameliorated and often eliminated by energy psychology approaches.

> Energy psychology methods are consistently effective for ongoing events, such as the complex relationship issues that caregivers are most often involved in.

How energy psychology techniques work

Energy psychology practitioners have discovered many forms of stimulation that can be applied to the meridians in order to adjust the movement of chi within and between the meridians. Various methods used to stimulate the flow of chi along the meridians include

- applying pressure on the acupoints with the fingers, which is called acupressure
- rubbing or tapping on the various acupoints
- running one's hand over the meridian in the direction of the flow of that meridian's chi.

As each meridian is stimulated, the chi circulating in the meridian system is mobilized, creating mental and emotional shifts at multiple levels. The underlying theory is that as you mobilize your vital force, your chi begins to return to a balanced state. There is an observable correlation between the harmony or disharmony of the circulating chi within us and the thoughts and feelings we are experiencing at any given time. Our thoughts and feelings are part of what some quantum physicists call "information fields" or energetic fields of influence associated with each meridian. When we become stressed or threatened, the flow of chi in one or more of our meridians becomes perturbed, which frequently creates mental and emotional imbalance. When these "thought fields" are discharged through the implementation of a meridian stimulation method, such as tapping or applying pressure on a meridian endpoint, the mental and/or emotional disturbance evaporates. As the chi in one or more meridians comes into balance, the information that created and maintained the disturbance is no longer circulating. Since the body, mind and spirit are integrally interconnected, restoring the balanced flow of chi through the meridians also changes our thoughts and feelings.

Since these shifts happen at the energetic level, the specific emotions connected to the meridians that were out of balance start to come back to homeostasis as negative emotional charge is released. Typical signs that a shift is happening during the meridian stimulation process include deep exhalations, sighing, yawning and an increasing and pervasive feeling of calm and physical relaxation.

> Since the body, mind and spirit are integrally interconnected, restoring the balanced flow of chi through the meridians also changes our thoughts and feelings.

An important component of these meridian-stimulating techniques is that the individual is directed to think about his problem or deliberately experience the stressful emotional state related to his problem while he is doing the meridian stimulation. This is referred to as an exposure-based therapeutic approach, and it generally results in the immediate and rapid alleviation of the client's problem state.

Dr. David Feinstein is a prominent researcher studying the effects of energy psychology interventions, most notably a tapping intervention called Emotional Freedom Techniques® or EFT. The following is an excerpt of his research:

> In energy psychology, as with other exposure-based treatments, exposure is achieved by eliciting—through imagery, narrative, and/or in-vivo [real-life] experience—hyperarousal associated with a traumatic memory or threatening situation. Unique to energy psychology is that extinction of this association is facilitated by 1) the manual stimulation of acupuncture and related points that are believed to 2) send signals to the amygdala and other brain structures that 3) quickly reduce hyperarousal. When the brain then reconsolidates the traumatic memory, the new association (to reduced hyperarousal or no hyperarousal) is retained. According to practitioners, this leads to treatment outcomes that are more rapid (less time; fewer repetitions) and more powerful (higher impact; greater reach) than the strategies used by other exposure-based treatments that are available to them, such as relaxation, desensitization, mindfulness, flooding, or repeated exposure. Another clinical strength reported by practitioners is increased precision, and thus less chance of retraumatization. By being able to quickly reduce hyperarousal to a targeted stimulus, numerous aspects or variations of a problem may be identified, precisely formulated, and treated within a single session.[2]

While the effectiveness of acupuncture treatments for physiological problems is well known (many health insurance companies now include and pay for acupuncture treatments), openness to these new and non-Western methods for treating psychological problems requires considering some ideas that are not yet accepted by mainstream Western psychiatry and psychology. After all, I am asking you to entertain the possibility that by simply tapping on meridian points on your face, chest and hands while staying connected to your problem state, immediate cognitive and emotional shifts will result. This is very different from the talk therapy methods that have dominated the Western approach to the treatment of emotional problems since Freud introduced psychoanalysis in the early 1900s.

Energy psychology tools for emergency situations

Now that you know about some of the basic principles that explain *why* your bioenergy system becomes unbalanced and disrupted, it's time to learn *how* to apply some easy-to-use, practical techniques you can begin using right now.

Please note that because these revolutionary techniques have only been in widespread use since the mid-1980s, they are still considered relatively new and innovative by practitioners of mainstream Western psychology, and are often viewed with some suspicion. The consensus among energy psychology practitioners is that it is not necessary to spend hours talking about and trying to analyze the underlying reasons for why you are experiencing certain symptoms of distress. These insights tend to emerge spontaneously as an epiphenomenon of applying these energy balancing strategies.

I invite you to be curious and try out the techniques discussed below so you can experience firsthand the inherent wonder and intelligence of your own self-healing capabilities. They're easy to use, they generate rapid and frequently immediate experiential shifts, and they can be used anywhere and anytime. By recruiting your own vital energy with these very specific techniques, you will boost your confidence and immediately start feeling better about yourself. More to the point, you will discover a consistently reliable way to extricate yourself from what previously felt like heavy and even hopeless emotional challenges.

> You will discover a consistently reliable way to extricate yourself from what previously felt like heavy and even hopeless emotional challenges.

While it's true that all of us need help and support from other people, prescription medications, and practitioners of Western psychiatry/psychology at certain times, deliberately and systematically recruiting your own energy-based self-healing capabilities provides a way for you to take more personal responsibility for maintaining your emotional equanimity by keeping your essential energy system balanced.

I have been clinically practicing, writing about and teaching energy psychology methods for nearly fourteen years. There are many different approaches to implementing energy psychology methods for emotional balance and well-being. Outlined below is an easy-to-follow protocol that you can begin using right now. I want to take you through this step-by-step, to give you yet another set of powerful self-care resources to draw upon in order to avoid the caregiver's inherent risk of secondary traumatization and burnout as you support and assist others.

Before you begin, make sure you are well hydrated. As I stated in Chapter 9, this is essential when you are systematically working with and balancing your vital energy system. I recommend that you keep drinking sufficient amounts of water while implementing these techniques.

Make sure your energy system isn't "switched"

Your first step is to ensure that your energy system is open and responsive to any of the energy balancing techniques that you are implementing. For this to happen, you must make sure that your bioenergy system is not switched; that is, you need to ensure that your system is ready and initially balanced so that you can be certain that your efforts will be successful!

Energy psychology practitioners have discovered that there are a variety of reasons for why your energy system can become scrambled and create a condition that is known as being switched. When this happens, your meridians literally begin to run backwards and your energy becomes reversed. When your energy is switched, you may

- experience mental or physical sluggishness, to the point of physically bumping into things
- become inarticulate, mixing up or forgetting words
- become forgetful
- feel spacy
- feel that you aren't connected to yourself
- just feel "off"

There are many possible reasons for why this may be occurring. A sensitivity reaction to a food that you've eaten, or to an environmental toxin such as gasoline or paint fumes, can throw off your energy system. Other times, the switch may result from overexposure to electromagnetic radiation in your environment. This can occur if you've been working around large machinery or engines, such as a leaf blower, chainsaw or lawnmower, or even if you have been sitting at a computer for many hours. Your energy can even become switched if you become emotionally upset or stressed to the degree that it reverses the energy flow in one or more meridians.

Since it is very difficult to know whether the way you are feeling is the result of any of these variables, or to know whether you are actually switched, it is important to be proactive and routinely use the following exercise as a way to ensure system readiness prior to implementing the energy psychology self-help strategies that follow.

While there are a number of ways to address this issue, one of the most straightforward and uncomplicated methods I've learned is Donna Eden's "three thumps."[3] By tapping the following three specific sets of points located on your body, you will become more energized—it gives your overall vitality a general pick-me-up—and more mentally focused. In addition, any meridians that were switched will usually come back into their normal directional flow, enabling a neutral starting point for the energy balancing techniques to follow. The three thumps strategy has also been determined to stimulate your immune system.

The first points to tap on are the twenty-seventh acupoints along the kidney meridians, which are located in the hollow areas

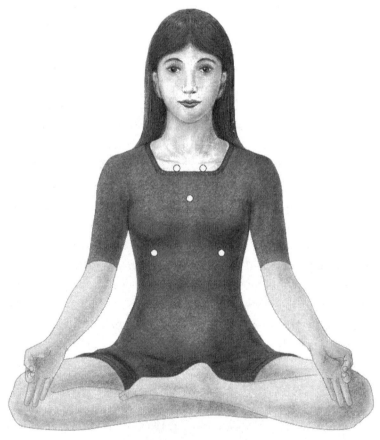

Three-thumps tapping points

just below your collarbones (the slight indent under the collar bones that most people have). Place your index and middle fingers next to each other. Cross your hands over each other so that your palms are facing your chest, the fingers on your right hand are tapping under your left collarbone, and the fingers on your left hand are tapping under your right collarbone. Tap or "thump" these points for approximately twenty seconds. Crossing your hands helps to enable your neuro-impulses to cross over from the right side of your brain to the left side of your body and from the left side of your brain to the right side of your body, which allows optimal communication of neurological impulses throughout your nervous system. This helps you access your brain's full potential because it elicits and sends information more effectively throughout your nervous system and physical body.

The next area to tap is over your thymus. It is located in the center of your chest, at the sternum bone. This is approximately two inches below the kidney points you just tapped. This time, use four fingers of either hand (it doesn't matter which hand) to tap on or thump your thymus point for about twenty seconds.

The last points to tap are the neurolymphatic points that are connected to your spleen meridian. These are approximately two inches below your breast. Using two or more fingers on each hand, tap or thump your spleen points for approximately twenty seconds. Many people find it awkward to cross their hands over while doing this, but it is fine to cross them over if you want to.

Once you have completed this three thumps tapping sequence, you are ready to move on to the next step, which is learning how to measure your own level of distress. You will use this technique to subjectively assess your current emotional state, and to keep track of how you are progressing as you use the tapping technique.

Use the SUDS rating scale

In 1958, Dr. Joseph Wolpe developed a self-rating scale that is based on subjective units of distress (SUDS). You assign a rating, on a scale of zero through ten, to your degree of inertia, frustration or distress relative to a specific issue you are presently experiencing. A zero rating indicates that you are feeling neutral, while a ten rating indicates the highest level of distress that you can imagine feeling.

Wolpe's SUDS self-rating scale is used in the field of psychology for all kinds of self-rating evaluations. It's extremely helpful as a way for you to stay focused and connected to a problem state that you're actively working on eliminating. I teach many of my clients how to follow their own SUDS level of disturbance while using the EFT tapping technique in my office. This gives them a powerful self-care tool to use at home or at their office whenever they feel it is necessary.

Use Emotional Freedom Techniques®

I would now like to teach you how to use Emotional Freedom Techniques® (EFT). This is a wonderful energy psychology technique that will help you with stress management and burnout prevention. First, some brief background about how EFT was developed.

Roger Callahan's Thought Field Therapy® is based on the idea that tapping on specific combinations of different meridian acupoints is effective in treating certain problems that Callahan has catalogued. For example, a particular sequence of tapping points, which Callahan called algorithms, is most helpful in alleviating phobias, while a different algorithm is most helpful in treating panic attacks.

A related technique was developed by Gary Craig, who was one of Callahan's first students. Craig found that clients could achieve results that were just as effective without having to memorize specific algorithms correlated to particular problems. He developed a procedure in which the client taps on the endpoints of ten of the twelve major meridians, and on the endpoints of the Governing and Central meridians. The Central and Governing meridians are not connected to any particular organ system, but the energies you encounter in your outer environment can circulate in and out of you through these two central meridians.[4] The Central meridian (sometimes called the Central vessel or Conception vessel) is located along the front of the body, connecting a point just below the lower lip to a point near the pubic bone. The Governing meridian (sometimes called the Governing vessel) starts just under the nose, goes up over the top of the head, and then straight down the back of the body to the very base of the spine. Craig called his approach Emotional Freedom Techniques®.

Energy psychology practitioners have since modified Craig's "basic recipe" in a variety of ways. The technique that I describe below is my modification of EFT, which involves tapping on all twelve of the major meridians plus the Governing and Central meridians. I have found that this modification provides a more comprehensive treatment approach. Illustrations 2a and 2b show which endpoints are tapped in my modified EFT technique.

Step 1: *Attunement*

After you have done all that you can to make sure that your energy system isn't switched, identify your initial SUDS level for the problem you're working on. This initial rating becomes your reference point for how emotionally stressed you are about the incident or issue, which you will refer back to as you work through the problem. To determine what initial rating to give yourself, consider what you are feeling (or what you are disturbed about) *at this moment.* Rate your feelings from zero to ten, with ten being "extremely distressed" and zero being "neutral."

Make a note of your initial SUDS rating in your journal so you have a record of it. As you work through the specific issue using EFT, write down what you become aware of after each sequence of tapping and to what degree your SUDS level changes. This helps you track your progress and identify each component that emerges during the EFT tapping process. If this same issue

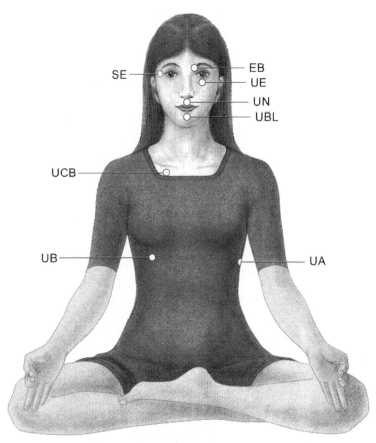

2a: EFT Points

or symptom comes up again in the future, you can refer back to your journal entries to compare what is the same and what, if anything, has changed. Additionally, journaling each new aspect of your unfolding awareness during your tapping will help you to stay focused on what you most need to pay attention to.

In the account of one marriage counselor's experience given earlier in this chapter, Carolyn felt threatened and emotionally upset after the abusive husband yelled at her with his finger inches away from her face. That experience occurred at the office during her workday, but it wasn't until she got home that night

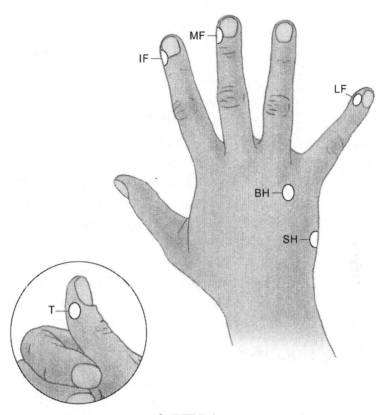

2b: EFT Points

that Carolyn had time to reflect and work on her feelings about the experience. At home that evening, she assigned herself a SUDS level of nine, meaning that at that moment in the evening, her stressful feelings about the earlier event were at a nine. She recorded this rating in her journal, for future reference. Note that the "earlier event" could just as easily have been something that happened last month, or even five years ago. The important point is that you rate how you are feeling about the issue or incident *now*, no matter how long ago it actually happened.

It is sometimes the case that a client continues to be disturbed by a past event and recognizes its continuing negative impact on his life right now. Sometimes the client's emotions are right on the surface and can be mobilized easily and quickly. In other cases, even though the client may be numb or dissociated and not feel anything at all, he continues to mentally obsess about the event or have ongoing intrusive memories of what occurred. Even if you are not *feeling* the emotional upset about the event, using EFT will be just as effective when you focus your attention on *thinking* about or remembering the upset. In fact, many energy psychology clinicians believe that for people with strong trauma-laden emotions just below the surface (that is, PTSD), it is actually therapeutically better to just *think* about the trauma. Re-experiencing the traumatic feelings associated with the event puts the individual at risk of being retraumatized and possibly overwhelmed by those powerful emotions while implementing EFT. The point is to bring your attention and awareness to the issue that is the disturbance in any focused way you can while tapping on the EFT points.

The next step is to keep your attention on the problem or the situation that is causing you inner conflict or distress as you begin tapping on the fourteen points used in my Dynamic Energetic Healing® adaptation of EFT. This is called *attunement*. As you are attuning to what is most prominent in your awareness about the problem *now*, you tap on each of the points in sequence, starting on the face, then on the trunk of the body, and finally on the fingers and hand.

Step 2: *Do the tapping*

The tapping procedure is done with the fingertips of the index and middle fingers together of whichever hand feels most comfortable for you. You tap on each acupoint six or seven times before moving on to the next one. The summary of the EFT treatment points given in the following table lists each meridian point and its abbreviation, followed by the name of the meridian and the particular emotions associated with that meridian.

EFT Treatment Points

Meridian Point	Part of Body Addressed	Emotions Addressed
Eyebrow (EB)	Bladder	Trauma, frustration
Side of eye (SE)	Gallbladder	Rage, resentment
Under eye (UE)	Stomach	Disgust, anxiety, nervousness
Under nose (UN)	Governing vessel	Fear of failure, embarrassment
Under bottom lip (UBL)	Conception vessel	Shame
Under collarbone (UCB)	Kidney	Fear, insecurity
Under arm (UA)	Spleen	Low self-esteem, insecurity
Under breast (UB)	Liver	Anger, unhappiness
Thumb (T)	Lung	Grief, arrogance
Index finger (IF)	Large intestine	Guilt, dogmatism
Middle finger (MF)	Pericardium	Jealousy, regret, cravings
Little finger (LF)	Heart	Anger
Side of hand (SH)	Small intestine	Loss, sadness, vulnerability
Back of hand (BH)	Triple warmer	Depression, cognitive confusion

Start by tapping at the base of your eyebrows (EB), followed by tapping on the side of your eyes (SE), and then under your eyes (UE). The next points are under your nose (UN), followed by under your bottom lip (UBL). These complete the points on the face.

Proceed to the points on the trunk of your body by tapping on the kidney points under your collarbones (UCB), followed by tapping four inches under your armpits (UA), and then just below your breasts (UB).

The last part of the sequence is done on the designated points on either hand. Start with the outside of your thumb by the fingernail (T), followed by the same side of your index finger by the fingernail (IF), your middle finger by the fingernail (MF), and your little finger by the fingernail (LF). Then tap the fleshy part of the side of the hand (SH), which is the same spot used to address psychoenergetic reversal (see Chapter 6). Complete the entire sequence by tapping on the back of your hand between the little finger and the ring finger (BH).

As you progress through the tapping sequence, just notice what comes up for you, such as a strong feeling, an inner conflict, a sensation of tightness somewhere in your body or perhaps even a memory connected to the event. Essentially, you are free associating and allowing whatever is in your awareness to be present in what becomes an organically driven unfolding process.

To illustrate how EFT tapping can help an individual caregiver, let's go back to the example of Susan the hospice worker. In Chapter 6, I outlined Susan's dilemma about reducing her workload by ten hours per week. There, I explained that, in her case, the first issue she had to deal with was her psychoenergetic reversal. To do that, she tapped the "karate-chop" point on the side of her hand while repeating the psychoenergetic reversal statement three times out loud.

Revisiting Susan

After Susan corrected her reversal, I asked her to self-rate any emotional charge about her dilemma using the SUDS scale. She gave her feeling of frustration related to not being able to follow through on her intention to work fewer hours a subjective rating of nine out of ten. Now it was time for her to go through my modified version of tapping the EFT points, starting on her face.

As Susan began the EFT tapping, she reflected on the *feeling* of inner conflict and the *confusion in her thinking* that continued to prevent her from making the decision that she wanted to make. In other words, she attuned to the elements that were causing her to feel frustrated and unable to comfortably choose to fulfill her true desire.

After Susan finished the fourteen-point tapping sequence, she paused to reflect on how she was feeling emotionally, what she was thinking about, and whether she was aware of any new sensations in her body. Following my recommendation that she journal her EFT tapping process, Susan wrote down her awareness of *feeling enormous guilt* for abandoning her clients, who are in great despair and need. She also wrote down that she was *feeling a knot in her stomach*. Reflecting on the SUDS self-rating scale again, she admitted to herself that even though she was experiencing this guilt and the physical symptom in her stomach, by focusing on her inner conflict she had actually lessened her anxiety about it. (This insight emerged spontaneously for Susan, with no prompting from me.) Susan decided that she had reduced the feeling of frustration about moving forward with her intention from a nine down to a seven. Although this rating change might seem minimal, she acknowledged that something was beginning to shift. At the same time, she was clear that she had much more to do before coming to a place of resolution about the issue. Susan made a note of this SUDS self-rating change in her journal.

Then, she immediately began her second round of EFT tapping. This time, she focused on (and attuned to) what Gary Craig has called the newly emerging *aspects* or foci of her unfolding awareness process. In Susan's case, that included feelings of guilt for abandoning her clients and the tension in her stomach. As she tapped each of the endpoints on her face, trunk and hands, she continued to bring all of her awareness to these feelings. To emphasize her attentional absorption during her tapping process, she said out loud, "Feeling guilty, knot in my gut" while tapping each point.

When Susan completed her tapping sequence for the second time, she again paused and reflected on what she was feeling emotionally, what she was thinking about, and any new sensations in her body. She even became aware of a memory that came to the surface completely uninvited. She remembered how she had felt guilty when, at 9 years old, she played with her friends outside after school instead of helping her mother care for her father, who had Parkinson's disease. By that time, Susan's father was quite disabled.

Because of Susan's inherent sensitivity, the guilt and inner conflict she felt *then* related to her mother and father was similar to the feelings she was currently experiencing with her own children and her clients.

Susan noticed that she suddenly felt much more relaxed than when she started the tapping process, and the sensation of tightness in her stomach had completely dissipated. Additionally, she no longer felt guilt about abandoning her clients. Instead, Susan noticed a *feeling of sadness*, which she related to not spending more time with her children. When she reflected once again on her SUDS self-rating scale, she rated her feelings at a three, and wrote this new information in her journal. She had made significant progress that time!

In what turned out to be her last EFT tapping sequence, Susan focused her attention on her feelings of sadness related to not spending more time with her children. At one point during this tapping sequence, she was aware that she let out a deep sigh, followed by a feeling of further physical relaxation.

After completing her third round of the tapping sequence, Susan realized that she felt calm and surprisingly resolute in her newly found knowledge about how important it felt to spend more time with her children. The tension in her body was gone, and she decided that she was at a zero on the self-rating scale. As is frequently the case when people try EFT for the first time, Susan was surprised at how quickly she resolved what had been tormenting her for weeks. She now felt absolutely congruent about her decision, and the conflicting thoughts (the cognitive dissonance) that had been preventing her from making a decision were resolved into one clear intention. She made some final notes in her journal, so she could refer to them in the future if her inner conflict about her children and her work ever arose again.

Susan's example reflects an energy-based self-care strategy of the highest order. While Susan experienced resolution of her problem in a relatively short time with only three repetitions of the EFT sequence, this does not always happen. Each person's situation is unique, and I could give you many clinical examples of more complicated problems that required more time, with many more emerging aspects that the client needed to focus on before the self-rating scale was finally reduced to a one or zero.

In some cases, clients who have reduced their SUDS numerical rating (such as working down from a nine to a six) suddenly hit a wall and perceive no more progressive movement down the self-rating scale, or even jump back up to an eight after completing a round of EFT tapping. When this occurs, the client has run up against a spontaneously occurring psychoenergetic reversal. This may be described as hitting a subconscious block that will not yield. In these cases, I direct clients to tap on the side of one hand (as described in Chapter 6), with a modified setup phrase to repeat three times: "I completely and profoundly accept myself *even though I have jumped from a six back up to an eight!*" The client then continues to tap on all the EFT treatment points while repeating the shortened focus phrase, "Jumped from a six to an eight." By the time they have completed tapping all fourteen points, they have usually corrected the psychoenergetic block and can then continue to progress on their issue from where they left off.

How effective is EFT?

While EFT is not a panacea, it often successfully resolves emotional and physical problems when nothing else has worked. Research among energy psychology practitioners suggests that EFT brings complete or partial relief in about 80 percent of the cases in which it's tried, and in the hands of a skilled practitioner, its success rate can exceed 95 percent.[5] Ongoing research reflects the effectiveness of EFT with different populations, including current studies on the success of EFT in the short-term treatment of Iraq war veterans with PTSD. The Andrade–Feinstein study tracked over 29,000 patients from eleven allied treatment centers in South America over a fourteen-year period. "In this study 90 percent of the experimental group (using tapping) improved, and 76 percent were judged to be symptom-free (as opposed to 63 percent and 51 percent of the control group, respectively)."[6]

EFT has been found to be effective for establishing energetic boundaries with aggressive individuals and alleviating symptoms of PTSD, specific phobias, depressed mood and panic attacks. Additionally, many people use EFT successfully to ameliorate and eliminate chronic and persistent physical problems, including migraine headaches, gastrointestinal problems and flu-like stress symptoms, all of which are common self-care challenges for high-intensity relaters.

> EFT has been found to be effective for establishing energetic boundaries with aggressive individuals and alleviating symptoms of PTSD, specific phobias, depressed mood and panic attacks.

Long-term problems require much greater persistence, especially when EFT is the only strategy being used. Some energy psychology practitioners use EFT as the only intervention or approach to assist their clients. Using only EFT with someone who is suffering from long-term PTSD or depression, for example, can be profoundly successful but it may take six to ten one-hour sessions to achieve significant reductions in the worst chronic symptoms of a disorder that had persisted for many years. In other situations involving long-term problems, EFT is just one of a number of tools that are used synergistically—along with other suggestions offered in this book—while collaborating with a healthcare professional. For instance, some of my clients have had to incorporate the regular use of EFT along with Bach flower remedies (see Chapter 8) and ongoing imagery techniques (see Chapter 11).

Self-care for high-intensity relaters requires effective, reliable techniques to bring their thoughts and emotions into balance quickly and then maintain that balance. Recruiting your essential energy system, which is circulating throughout your body (where all of your meridians are interconnected and even interact with the more highly concentrated energy fields of your chakras), *is something you can learn to do easily with astounding and immediate results.* This is true whether your symptoms of distress are the result of the everyday stressors that seem to come with the territory of high-intensity caregiving, or whether you are experiencing more serious and intense trauma-related issues. Regardless of the stressors that you are dealing with in your life right now, I encourage you to spend some time becoming familiar with tapping EFT points for resolving specific problem states, and with the many other energy psychology modalities that are widely available. (For more information about other energy psychology modalities, see pages 177–238 of my book *Dynamic Energetic Healing®*.) It is my fervent hope that EFT will be a good fit for you as a regular self-care strategy, and that you will find it to be very good medicine indeed.

> Recruiting your essential energy system, which is circulating throughout your body (where all of your meridians are interconnected and even interact with the more highly concentrated energy fields of your chakras), is something you can learn to do easily with astounding and immediate results.

Questions and Exercises

1. Once you have tried the techniques described in this chapter, consider making a list of all the *significant* hurts and traumatic events you can remember, going all the way back to your early childhood if you can. Then, identify the five events that you believe have been the worst or most stressful in your life. Think carefully about each event to determine whether

there is any negative emotional charge still lingering about this event. Does it bother you to have to think about the events? Would you be comfortable talking about the event to a friend or partner? Do you notice any tightening up in your body or distracting feeling states when you recall the event? Catalog your responses. If there is any residual trauma or negative emotional charge, your self-care will likely be sabotaged. Make a commitment to yourself to do what is necessary to eliminate these residual feelings, which can be described as traumatic residue.

2. Follow the procedures outlined in this chapter to clear away any traumatic residue associated with each of the five events you identified above. In summary,
   a) Drink some water.
   b) Establish system readiness.
   c) Correct for any psychoenergetic reversal.
   d) Establish your starting SUDS level on the issue.
   e) Go through the EFT protocol.
   f) After each sequence of tapping all the points, pause and reflect on what you notice, how you are feeling, what you are thinking and what kind of feedback your physical body is generating. Journal your responses.
   g) Continue with the EFT process until you have reduced your SUDS level down to a one or a zero.

   Consider making a commitment to spend thirty to sixty minutes every night working through all of your old hurts and traumas in this way until you have essentially zeroed out all residual negative emotional charge that you have been carrying as heavy emotional baggage. You can make the time to do it because you are worth it.

3. Now that you've cleared out these lingering traumas from your past, it will be much easier for you to stay current with

anything that confronts you in your day-to-day activities supporting others. If you don't clear out the significant traumas from your past that remain unhealed, you risk having one of your clients trigger or restimulate old traumatic residue that will compromise your effectiveness as a caregiver or helper. If this happens, it can set you up for secondary traumatization.

4. If you are unable to meet this self-care goal of detraumatizing yourself based on past events, consider consulting with a trained energy psychology practitioner who can help you.

CHAPTER

11

Making It Happen From Within

In recent chapters, I have discussed self-care strategies that include how to confront your inner critic, protect yourself from energy vampires, practice saying NO whenever necessary, and use the healing energies of plants and the natural world to release negative emotional charge and come back to a state of balance. EFT and the implementation of energy psychology tools are also valuable and easy to access self-care tools that will support you to prevent self-sabotage. In addition, teaching your clients how to use these tools will enable them to maintain a sense of control in their lives. This repertoire of powerful tools is designed to support your ongoing health and well-being, and to promote healthy chi management in all areas of your life as a high-intensity relater. While I use and recommend them all, it is the creative application of your imagination using imagery and structured exercises that I am particularly excited about sharing with you now. This inward focus supports your inherent genius to create a lifestyle that will best support your work and your life as you support others. I call this "making it happen from within."

> This inward focus supports your inherent genius. I call this "making it happen from within."

You can make positive and transformative changes in your life by going within yourself to consider ways of creating the best and most fulfilling life you can imagine. You begin by using your analytical, decision-making left brain to identify and prioritize your self-care goals. Following this, the right side of your brain also becomes activated as you imagine and visualize possibilities for how you would love to live your life as a high-intensity relater in the very near future, as expressed in your intention statements.

In Chapter 4, I discussed the fact that our thoughts (and prayers) affect others, whether we realize it or not. In this chapter, I want to focus on how you can use your thoughts and your imagination to make positive changes in your life that will support your self-care so you can stay optimally healthy.

The power of your intention

You may not be consciously aware that you are the ongoing creator of your life. This statement challenges the belief that everything that happens in your life is random. Simply through your thinking, you can create and draw into your life nearly anything you want. In essence, whatever you create always starts with a thought form or an idea.

In the emerging science of quantum physics, the self has a field of influence on the world and vice versa. At the subatomic level, what has been named the Zero Point Field is characterized as a state of pure potential and infinite possibilities. Every molecule and every living thing has a unique frequency that is constantly exchanging information in this quantum field of mutual influence. Quantum theory, partly based on subatomic particle experiments, repeatedly points to the influence of what we are thinking as determining outcomes for ourselves. The inference is that we affect our future simply by observing or intending it.

Let's start on the practical level: "I want to plant a garden this spring." What follows that thought are the actions required to make this intention happen, including measuring the space, identifying soil amendments and ordering the seeds. "I want to make seafood paella this weekend." I subsequently find myself making a shopping list, buying the fish, saffron and Spanish rice, and excitedly looking forward to preparing it. So it goes—thought precedes action and manifestation.

In these two examples, I have a strong desire to follow through on my initial thought because gardening and cooking paella are very gratifying to me. I create a new garden every spring and I make paella frequently. Thus, not only do I have a strong desire, but I also *know* that I can create the outcome of my initial thought or intention because I've done it before. But even if you have never accomplished what your initial desire or idealized goal is, you can start right now by thinking about new possibilities, and then nurturing your thinking to evolve into a more complex imaginative process or vision. While it may strike you as implausible that you can attain your self-care goals simply by imagining that you have achieved them, I know from my own experience that this is the way our universe works. Everyone is capable of this—in fact, everyone is doing this all the time, albeit usually not consciously. This is one of those universal truths that has always existed in every culture and civilization from time immemorial.

To convince you that you too can successfully implement these ideas and make them concrete, let me begin by disabusing you of a widely held belief that only a small percentage of people are able to use their creativity to become "successful" in the world. We give this small coterie of "creative individuals" celebrity status—they gain a worldwide following and the admiration of millions due to their success at creating significant accomplishments. Most notably, these creative individuals are accomplished in the performing arts, Nobel laureates across various disciplines, athletes with multimillion dollar contracts, and young entrepreneurs in the high-tech industry who create companies such as Apple, eBay, Amazon and Google. We tend to believe that these creative individuals are intellectually gifted and extraordinarily talented.

It would be overly simplistic to identify just one characteristic that led to these individuals' ultimate success. However, I am certain that each of them has been able to sustain an unwavering preoccupation and commitment to doing everything necessary to unfold their vision until it became actualized in form. In Chapter 2, I referred to Gardner's theory on multiple intelligences, in which he describes that some of us have propensities and inclinations that, if followed, will predict a greater degree of success in that area of our pursuit.

The exciting truth is that *everyone* can learn to do this!

Brain neuroplasticity and repetition

Neuroscientists have shown that our thoughts can affect other people. Amazingly, they have also shown that where we focus our attention and what we continually think about is what we become neurologically. New evidence from functional brain scans supports this conclusion. For example, a part of the brain called the hippocampus is measurably larger in London taxicab drivers than in a control group who are not cab drivers.

> Black Cab drivers are renowned for being ultra-brainy: they are expected to memorise the route of up to 250,000 different roads in the capital, and they are not given a licence until they have demonstrated they have "The Knowledge" ... Scientists have now discovered that cab drivers have an internal Satnav [satellite navigational system], that many of us do not have, and it has been located in the hippocampus towards the back of the brain. Cab drivers were found to have an enlarged hippocampus which started firing neurons like mad as their cab driver owners ruminated on what route to take from A to B.
>
> "The hippocampus is crucial for navigation and we use it like a 'sat nav'," Dr. Hugo Spiers of the Institute of Behavioural Neuroscience at UCL told the BA Festi-

val of Science in Liverpool today. "London taxi drivers have powerful innate satnavs, strengthened by years of experience."[1]

The study above challenges the older neuroscience paradigm that our brains are hardwired from birth. As a result of repeatedly focusing their attention on learning the labyrinthine London streets, the brain tissue of these cab drivers grew and changed. This is called neuroplasticity.

This concept in neuroscience is called Hebbian learning. The idea is simple: nerve cells that fire together wired together. Therefore, when gangs of neurons are repeatedly stimulated, they will build stronger, more enriched connections between each other.[2]

Any of us can do what the London cabbies are able to do. Using creative visualization and imagery in a way that is focused, disciplined and repeated frequently actually rewires your brain by engaging circuits that process associated sensory stimulation. For the brain to forge stronger neurological connections, it matters little what activity you're practicing. Your brain will grow the more you repeat an action, the more you reinforce a thought and the more energy and attention you provide to the given activity. Focused attention is a skill you develop through your ongoing commitment to the task at hand. This is all about repetition! *Successful outcomes from any activity you're working toward gaining proficiency in have to be practiced or repeated frequently.* This is why mentally rehearsing one's imagined positive outcome for a self-care goal is so very important.

> *Successful outcomes from any activity you're working toward gaining proficiency in have to be practiced or repeated frequently.*

We must fall in love with this vision, never tiring of, or becoming bored by, this concept of ourselves. We are all a work in progress. We should always feel that we want to be with our new concept and visit with it. We must bond with a pattern of thinking that repeatedly inspires, enlivens, and heals us.[3]

Visualize to access the infinite

One of the most surprising and healing benefits of creative visualization is how consistently people describe spontaneously and unexpectedly perceiving the boundless and the ineffable, a state of consciousness that is sometimes called the Higher Self.

Some scientists theorize that these experiences could be related to the activation of the temporal lobes, which have been associated with perceptions of spiritual realities, but it's not just the activation of the temporal lobes that creates these perceptions of the numinous. Exciting new research using functional brain scans reveals that different parts of the brain are stimulated through different visualization and spiritual practices. These studies also show that the person who is visualizing or praying has a corresponding experience of their infinite nature, depending on what part of the brain is being activated.[4]

These spontaneous experiences tend to open the heart to feelings of love and greater openness, which is often experienced as a personal connection to God or Goddess, Greater Intelligence, departed and wise ancestors, guardian angels, and the souls of great teachers and masters from all the great religious traditions. What's interesting to me is that regardless of how each of us conceptualizes or experiences this subjective spiritual reality, it can be found and revealed within each of us right here and right now. What's more, the language and the imagery that describe these profound interior experiences frequently support the individual's particular religious teachings—the spontaneous experiences complement and augment a person's existing spiritual connection and beliefs.

Based on my many years of practicing hypnotherapy and imagery techniques, I would say that as clients move their rational left brain out of the way to open up to their subconscious mind, they're stepping into the doorway that puts them in direct contact with their Higher Self or Universal Mind, of which our own mind is just a part. When this contact is made, their spiritual nature is activated and their heart begins to open. While many questions remain about just how visualization and imagery work, innovative doctors have been researching its healing effects on the human body and illness for decades now.

You can heal yourself with imagery

In the 1970s, Dr. O. Carl Simonton and his wife, Stephanie Matthews-Simonton were on the vanguard of the growing field of psychoneuroimmunology. In their 1975 article "Belief Systems and Management of Emotional Aspects of Malignancy," O. Carl Simonton commented that

> I have not found any patient [who showed spontaneous remission of cancer symptoms, or unexpectedly good responses] that did not go through a similar visualizing process. It might be a spiritual process. God healing them, up and down the whole spectrum. But the important thing was what they pictured in the way they saw things. They were positive, regardless of the source, and the picture was very positive.[5]

The Simontons' research showed that when properly motivated, a patient's creative visualization could discover the cause of his or her own cancer and create the cure for it. When the patient generates the appropriate imagery, their body's immunological response is stimulated into destroying even the most widespread malignancies. This ability is within every one of us.

How visualization works

Creative visualization processes fall into a number of different categories. These include

- *programmed visualization*, which involves specific mental rehearsal that focuses on a particular goal or end result,
- *open-ended and receptive visualization*, such as contemplating how your life will be different and what new things you'll be doing when, for example, you have a lot more extra time because you've cut down on your working hours, and
- *guided imagery*, such as a guided meditation that you listen to on CD. These usually begin with progressive relaxation, and then continue to describe and direct you, step by step, to imagine a specific scenario that you can revisit in the same way many times.

Even though these approaches are distinct, in practice it's likely that they will overlap, as illustrated in the scenario described below.

To gain the maximum benefit from using any of these visualization techniques,

- You must have a clear goal in mind.
- You must mentally rehearse an intended outcome by visualizing it repeatedly.
- You must involve both hemispheres of your brain during your visualization. To do this, you recruit all of your faculties (seeing, hearing, smelling, tasting, and touching) to create visualizations that include as much sensory detail as possible. Neuroscience has shown that by doing this, you are actually switching on more groupings of neurons in your brain than when you're just using words.

But how does visualizing actually help you to attain a goal? Functional brain scan experiments continue to confirm that during mental rehearsal,

> the brain does not know the difference between what it is thinking (internal) and what it experiences (external). . . . In other words, in mental rehearsal, we change our brain before the external experience happens, and the brain is no longer a record of the past, but of the future.[6]

Essentially, you're synching your conscious intentions with your subconscious mind so that, eventually, you don't have to put so much mental effort into making something happen in your everyday experience. Through accessing deeper brain states by entering into the subconscious realm, you are connecting to that interior place where your habits and subsequent behaviors are formed and eventually solidify. One might say that this is the realm where lasting change happens. Because of the way your imagination becomes stimulated while you visualize, it's likely that your interior experience is going to be anything but linear. Memories associated with what you are visualizing will be triggered spontaneously. In addition, as more neural networks become stimulated, you will experience more simultaneous whole-brain processing. You can't know exactly *how* your goal is going to actualize, only that it will in what will probably be an unexpected and exciting unfolding.

Visualization and imagery for improving memory

You access different parts of your brain comprehensively and simultaneously when you are visualizing. Experiments show that, as a result, accessing and integrating new information through visualization makes it more likely that your memory will be significantly improved than if you used only the rational, thinking part of your brain. I know from personal experience that this is true.

In 1982, I was practicing hypnotherapy and studying how our subconscious beliefs affect our outer life. In my research, I came across *Super-Learning*.[7] This book is full of exercises for improving study skills, learning new information and remembering the new material almost effortlessly and more effectively than the normal approach we take. The aim of the exercises is to stimulate the imagination by using rich imagery, fantasy and positive affirmations. The technique also involved listening to music from the classical period (Mozart's era) while studying, which is also known as the Mozart effect. I wanted to test these approaches experimentally.

With the permission of my older son's third grade teacher, I came into the classroom for one hour twice a week for twelve weeks. My visits were dedicated to spelling, since students' progress in this area would be easy to quantify. The teacher gave me the names of the students and their average grade on spelling tests from the previous twelve weeks. She and I explained to the class that my research in hypnosis and storytelling led me to teach a very different way to master spelling words. Naturally, my son was totally stricken that his father was up in front of his class describing what seemed like a pretty hokey proposal. But he learned over time that this just came with the territory of having me as his father!

At the beginning of each week, we went over the twenty spelling words for that week, spelling them out as the students followed along on their spelling list at their desk. Next, I narrated imaginative and very silly stories. Initially, as the students and I were still getting comfortable with one another, I read short stories from *Put Your Mother on the Ceiling: Children's Imagination Games*.[8] These were goofy fantasy vignettes designed to stimulate children's imagination by leading them to visualize improbable fantasies. It got the children laughing and relaxed, until eventually I was able to free-associate to create my own silly stories.

At that time, I was taking extensive training in a subspecialty of hypnotherapy called Ericksonian hypnosis. I learned that all language is hypnotic because we must go inside ourselves to make sense of and decode the verbal communication being sent to us. As a consequence, we're always in a state of relative inter-personal trance or attentional absorption when we are interacting with others. Through the use of embedded metaphors and other techniques particular to storytelling and indirect suggestion, I learned about the power of words to create internal imagery and altered states of consciousness specific to supporting my clients to elicit powerful healing responses during a hypnosis session. I also learned how to trust this kind of extemporaneous story-telling that put *me* in an altered state of heightened creativity.

The kids just cracked up and thought I was totally off the wall and ridiculous, but they were completely caught up in the power of story, experiencing in their imagination a fantasy reality that I was shaping with my words.

There was a strategic reason for starting off this way. First, I was helping the students to think in images rather than words. This was turning on neural networks that would normally not be engaged by just trying to memorize the spelling words by rote. Second, I was helping the students relax and laugh, thus dissipating any tension or anxiety about learning that they might have been carrying.

Establishing deep relaxation so that the mind and body are calmed and quieted is essential for effective visualization in any context. Whether you're practicing a sitting meditation for thirty minutes or visualizing by mentally rehearsing the outcome of a self-care goal you are intending to carry out, if your body or mind is distracting you, your ability to maintain mental focus and your ultimate outcome are significantly compromised. Stretching, walk-ing or yogic deep breathing exercises are all ways to move out nervous tension from the body *prior* to sitting down for a session of creative visualization. So getting the kids to laugh at my silly stories was intentional for all the reasons above.

I interspersed positive affirmations throughout the stories, both directly and indirectly, as a way to further relax and encourage the students to be successful at easily learning their spelling words for the week. When the imagination games and the storytelling were over, I asked all the students to close their eyes and put their head down on their desk while I played various Mozart pieces from my cassette tape player and spelled out each of the words until I had completed the entire list. This was followed by the kids taking out their spelling list again as we spelled out each word one more time until we were done.

We went through the above process at the beginning of each week, and then repeated it on the day of the spelling test. With the exception of one boy who the teacher identified as dealing with some significant emotional problems, all the students in the class improved their spelling score by a least one grade! The students weren't particularly impressed by this because they were just having fun. But the teacher was awed, and we both felt enormously affirmed by how this very different paradigm for learning and memory was consistently successful.

This is a wonderful example of how significantly cognitive learning and memory can be enhanced by recruiting imagery and the gifts of the right cerebral hemisphere. If you are supporting parents or other seniors who are showing signs of dementia or memory decline, using some of the strategies outlined above could be a very helpful and supportive part of your caregiving. For example, play some soothing Mozart CDs softly as you read poems or stories that are rich in imagery. Stop occasionally to intersperse suggestions that your parent can remember what they need to whenever it is important.

For your own self-care, you could also consider acquiring some guided imagery CDs for specific personal issues you need some help with (such as insomnia or anxiety). Most of these CDs are accompanied with soothing music. For example, Belleruth Naparstek, who has written much about emotional trauma,[9] has developed a large catalog of healing CDs that the Department of Veterans Affairs is now using to help returning veterans heal from PTSD.

Guided imagery is so powerful because it can bypass our rational, thinking intellect to get to the parts of us that are more accessible to feelings and sensations, which is where much of the negative emotional charge resides.

The visualization techniques discussed in this chapter use right-brain strategies for actualizing your self-care goals. I want to just note that prior to engaging in any visualization process for your desired outcome, I recommend that you make an effort to consider and address specific psychoenergetic reversal that could interfere with your ability to actualize your self-care goals successfully. Psychoenergetic reversal and how to eliminate it (which is about preventing self-sabotage) is discussed in Chapter 6.

Step 1: Identify your goals
Think deeply about what you want
The starting point for using visualization as a self-care tool is to articulate what your self-care goals are. To help you start thinking, here are some categories of self-care goals you may want to consider:

- Create a manageable schedule that allows you to be in control of your day.
- Follow a specific exercise and dietary regimen that provides you with ongoing energy and excellent physical health, now and into the future.
- Create an evening ritual that supports you to sleep deeply through the night so you can wake up in the morning feeling rested and rejuvenated.
- Maintain a positive, upbeat mood while regularly interacting with people who are needy, traumatized and angry.
- Establish time in your life outside of work for activities that you find nurturing, fun and restoring, whether it be a daily qigong or meditation practice, or weekend excursions out of town to a special place that helps you feel you can still have adventures without having to get on a plane.

While I'm sure that you have numerous other personal goals that relate to promoting excellent self-care, you may find it helpful to use these broad categories to get you thinking about these topics. Depending on your disposition and clarity, you may be able to write out these statements of intention in ten minutes. On the other hand, you may need to spend a greater part of the weekend musing and reflecting on what it is you truly want in your life and what self-care issues are particularly pressing for you.

Be specific

Identifying your goals in general terms is just the first step—to actualize them, you must know *exactly* what you want! After working as a psychotherapist and group facilitator for over thirty years, I have learned that when people express their healing desires and intentions, they often don't think beyond their very general goal statements. For example, depressed people often say that their goal is to "no longer be depressed." Many overweight people express that their goal is to "lose weight." Those who are lonely say their goal is to "have a relationship."

These statements are good starting points, but you should be able to identify explicit details of what it would be like to, for example, no longer be depressed, or be in a relationship. Knowing exactly what you want with as much detail as possible must be your starting point.

So, take some time now to choose two of your most important self-care goals related either to your personal or professional life. To avoid getting discouraged, start off with short-term goals that you believe will be easily realizable. Write these out in as much detail as you possibly can.

Before proceeding to the next step, look within yourself to confirm whether you truly are 100 percent behind your goal and excited about its successful outcome. You have to be absolutely congruent about knowing what you want.

Step 2: Use a vision board to concretize your vision

If you are having difficulty visualizing your specific goal, don't give up. There is a powerful technique that will help you maintain and energize a sustained, focused image for optimizing the realization of your most important self-care goals.

Once you have identified and prioritized your personal goals for self-care, engaging your imagination with as much clarity as possible is essential. A well-known approach for supporting a positive outcome of a specific intention is a *vision board*. It's called this because you're constructing a physical picture or map of your desired new reality. A vision board is similar to a blueprint for a new building, and it is an invaluable way to jump-start your visualization process by creating particularly clear and sharp images.

> You have to be absolutely congruent about knowing what you want.

There are a variety of ways that you can construct this map. If you feel inspired or are creative in the visual arts, you can draw or paint your blueprint, either by hand or digitally (using software programs and importing clip art). But you don't have to identify yourself as a creative artist in order to do this well. You can create a collage in pictures and phrases (which will activate *both* sides of your brain) simply by buying as large a poster board as your space permits and collecting old or new interesting magazines, greeting cards and even photographs. Cut out pictures and phrases that speak to you, and tape them to your poster board. Keep your theme in mind, and include the phrases and pictures that reflect your vision.

For example, if insomnia is a self-care issue for you, choose pictures and phrases that reflect calm, nurturing relaxation. Images might include someone sleeping in a bed, lying on a chaise longue by a swimming pool in a resort, or floating on their back on the ocean in Hawaii or the Dead Sea. All of the pictures you select should bring you joy and instill a feeling of peacefulness. Associated phrases might be "My body and mind are in agreement now for sleeping deeply," "Sleep is balm to my soul" and "I feel safe in my home and easily drift into a deep sleep."

Place your vision board prominently somewhere in your home—for example, in your bedroom, bathroom or family room—where you will see it regularly. Being able to access it easily is essential. Just make sure that it won't be in the way of anyone else you are living with. Ideally, spend time with it first thing upon awakening and just before going to bed in the evening. Every time you see or glance at your vision board, your subconscious mind is being seeded. While this is just one piece in a larger process, the constant visual cues accompanying your ongoing mental focus (as previously described) will continue to bypass your thinking brain's resistance to create and experience your new reality.

> Every time you see or glance at your vision board, your subconscious mind is being seeded.

Can you have more than one vision board being implemented at any given time? Of course you can! Just consider for a moment how much information you are taking in every day all the time. Through various forms of multimedia such as television, movies, smart phones and the internet, you are constantly bombarding your nervous system and brain with enormous amounts of information. Creating one or more vision boards is a way of being intentionally discriminating by focusing your attention on specific information that you're absorbing for a clearly defined self-care outcome. By referring to your vision board, you're editing out or restricting input from everything that doesn't serve your present purpose as you are attending to your imagery.

Sitting in front of your vision board and reflecting on your clearly articulated and pictured goal will start to generate spontaneous connections and memories that will increase your internal network of positive associations related to your intention. This is not unlike classical meditation, in which a particular image is focused on for hours in an effort to deeply internalize a potent symbol of spiritual regeneration or liberation. In addition, speculating with "what if" questions will stimulate even more positive associations. For example, "What would it be like if I slept for seven hours straight?" "How much more would I be able to accomplish if I slept through the night?" "How would my mood be more positive during the day if I woke up feeling rested and energized?" As you reflect on these possibilities, you are imagining potential positive futures that previously had not been allowed due to your persistent insomnia. We all tend to stay preoccupied with a problem that prevents new possibilities from emerging. While you will likely still have to deal with some resistance to change from inside yourself, new ideas and possibilities are beginning to occupy more of your relationship with sleep. This gradual transition to "greater possibility thinking" becomes more automatic and internalized with any goal you choose to work on using these imagery-related techniques.

I lived in Los Angeles before moving to Oregon in 1977. Since I could not find work as a college teacher at that time in L.A., I decided to purchase a small acreage in Oregon in order to experience a different lifestyle. As I was researching various small acreage farming possibilities at the UCLA library, I purchased a book that became my guide for what is required to buy a home in the country. On the front cover of this very large book was a beautiful color photograph of an idealized rural property with beautiful trees and fields, and a creek running through the middle of it. Though I didn't know it at the time, this became my map or vision board for the property I was eventually to purchase. When I finally got settled in Oregon and the time came to begin looking for properties, I placed an offer on a beautiful fifteen-acre parcel on the western edge of the Willamette Valley.

When my offer was finally accepted, I was shocked to hear from my realtor that there had been eight other people interested in buying the property. To me, this reinforces how powerfully I was holding my vision of that country property. After all, it was a very desirable one, and perhaps it was only because I had such a persistently strong vision that I was able to prevail over eight others who were just as enthusiastic as I was to buy it. This experience makes me reflect on how, as the engaged "observer," I was continually influencing the outcome in my favor. It makes me question the whole notion of randomness.

To my utter delight and amazement, I realized that this property was virtually identical to the one shown on the front cover of the book that I had been studying for over two years. My subconscious mind had made it happen from within, in some mysterious and wonderful way, enabling me to be at the top of the list and in exactly the right place at the right time to make the first offer and have it accepted. Somehow, I had been able to hold the vision (with the help of the photograph on the book that I was assiduously internalizing on a daily basis) that manifested in my outer reality.

In fact, my vision was so strong that two years later I found an original oil painting by a local artist that appeared to be *my* beautiful rural property. It included the large pole barn, the old farmhouse, many beautiful blossoming trees and, of course, the creek running through the middle of the fifteen-acre property. This painting now hangs in the treatment room of my office as a personal reminder of the power of my intention to pursue things that are worthwhile and important.

Buying an acreage in Oregon was a vision that I was truly in love with, and I lived with it constantly for years before it finally came to fruition. I have had many other personal experiences of important goals manifesting in my life when *I was feeling very strongly* about how important they were for my well-being, happiness and self-care.

Step 3: Initiate your conscious dreaming process
Now that you have a clear understanding of what your specific goals are, the next step is to *engage your creative imagination to*

start "dreaming" about it and envisioning what the outcome will be.
The process I am outlining is just a more conscious and deliberate type of daydreaming, which everybody does. Imagine seeing yourself in the situation having already accomplished your goal. Imagine your objective already attained as you create the vision of yourself in the present time rather than at some undetermined time in the future. Aspects of this creative visualization process access and recruit

> Imagine seeing yourself in the situation having already accomplished your goal.

inner resource states saturated with rich fantasy accompanied by all the senses that are part of your normal everyday experience.

As you will see from the example below, this type of inner work puts you into a kind of trance, which is a state in which you become deeply attentionally absorbed. Therefore, you need to create some time and a space when and where you will not be interrupted. Even if you only spend three minutes doing this, your conscious dreaming process will yield results, but it demands your focused attention.

Example: Visualizing eating more vegetables
While *creative visualization* is widely recognized as integral to internal goal setting and the creation and manifestation of your desired outcomes, researchers have determined that only about 55 percent of the general population has a strong predisposition to easily visualize.[10] However, as the following hypothetical visualization scenario shows, imagery was only one part of the whole visualization experience.

Let's suppose that your goal is to increase your vegetable intake by 50 percent to experience greater physical energy. Part of your creative visualization or intentional dreaming process might include seeing yourself with your partner at a gourmet vegetarian restaurant—one that you have visited before, or that you are only now imagining. You might bring in your internal auditory channel by hearing yourself and your partner discussing which menu items sound most delectable and enticing. If you have eaten there before, try to remember some of the menu items that most interested you. If you've never eaten there before, you have to imagine, based on the very brief description of each menu item, what's going to be most appealing and will taste the best to you.

Your next inner vision could be of your server delivering to your table four exquisitely prepared dishes that smell delicious. At this point, you might ask yourself, "Is there a Middle Eastern, Thai, Japanese or Chinese restaurant I have been to before where I recall specific vegetarian entrées that left me amazed at how well vegetables can be prepared?" As your inner scenario continues to expand, bring all of your senses into play—the wonderful aromas, the appearance of the entrées, the texture as you crunch into the food, and the taste and temperature as the sensations spread across your tongue and create a sense of delight.

As this deeply immersive, multisensory fantasy continues to expand, you may notice your thoughts shifting from a familiar experience to wondering about new possibilities that you've never really given much thought to. For instance, you could think about all the different ways that you've enjoyed carrots and consider whether you can see yourself preparing and eating some of them, such as steamed carrots dribbled with olive oil and balsamic vinegar; freshly quartered carrots dipped into hummus or artichoke crab dip; carrot salad with raisins, jicama and a squeeze of lemon; freshly squeezed carrot juice (surprisingly sweet!); and, of course, a piece of carrot cake.

You might then shift to see in your mind's eye how all the vegetables are arranged in your local grocery store, and recall which vegetables you've considered buying but haven't yet. You might go through a process of elimination by *acknowledging to yourself verbally* that you've really never liked brussels sprouts (as you *feel yourself walking* by each area of the produce section, *picking up and handling* each of the vegetables *as you bring them one by one up to your nose for a smell*), but then you realize that artichokes, asparagus, broccoli and red onions have always appealed to you. Suddenly, a spontaneous memory pops up of the wonderful *warm feelings* of being nurtured by your grandparents during summertime picnics. They used to pick ears of corn right from their garden, throw them into the pots of boiling water, slather them with butter, and then pass an ear to you with those little plastic holders (yellow and shaped like a little ear of corn) on each end of the cob so your hands wouldn't get all greasy with butter.

Notice that as you continue to be immersed in this scenario, not only are you visualizing but you're engaging your kinesthetic, feeling and olfactory perceptual channels, which deepens the immersive experience. This is ideal, because the deeper you go into the experience of the visualization, the more you are priming the pump for the action plan that will follow. Then, out of the blue, you remember that a good friend has been a vegetarian for a number of years and has been inviting you over for a vegetarian dinner. She wants to share with you her latest tofu stir-fry recipe with a vegetable you've never tasted called bok choy.

> The deeper you go into the experience of the visualization, the more you are priming the pump for the action plan that will follow.

Note that this "eating more vegetables" visualization scenario is an example of programmed visualization. At the same time, it includes elements of open-ended/receptive daydreaming, since new ideas and memories arise as you focus on your goal of eating more vegetables. This example uses very detailed and vivid imagery, but it also shows that *visualization* need not be limited to imagery only. This scenario included *touching* and handling produce, *smelling* it, *physically moving* from one area of the produce section to the next, *hearing* inner conversations, and the *spontaneous recollection* of memories that are associated with the specific theme. The more you consciously engage your ability to visualize creatively, the more you expand and stimulate your whole-brain activation for making it happen from within. This repetitive imprinting of your inwardly created template in your mind soon begins to influence your outer world. You will notice that synchronicities happen to you more frequently—that is, the things that you only imagined will start to happen in your "real," external everyday life. It is through the power of your intent that you become a conscious artist; your own life is the canvas.

Next, I want to share with you three other visualization techniques that I'm sure will be helpful in your self-care.

Visualization Technique 1: Becoming your vision

In this approach, you visualize your desired completed action (for example, leaving your workplace at 5 PM instead of working late into the evening), and then visualize yourself *merging with* this completed action.[11]

Once you are absolutely clear about what your self-care goal (your desired completed action) is, imagine the completed action contained within a large white circle. You may be able to condense the circle to what you imagine to be just twelve inches across, or you may want the circle to be the size of your bedroom or your office. Take a moment to assess how large your circle is in your mind's eye.

The next step is to open up all the pores of your body and imagine yourself being filled up with the life-giving force of the Universal Intelligence or Higher Self with every inhalation, flooding into every part of you. See this life-giving force as a specific color; whatever color comes to you in your mind's eye is the appropriate color for you. Whether you see the color of the radiant sun or the sparkling azure of the Caribbean Sea, see and feel the energy from the Universal Intelligence filling you up with every breath you take, so that you become this growing globe of pulsating light. Take at least two or three minutes—or even longer—until you feel completely charged and saturated with this life-giving force of the Universal Intelligence.

When you feel and see yourself radiantly glowing and emanating this colored light from within, visualize your now radiant self merging with the circle that contains your completed action. At this point *you become the completed action*, infusing the circle with the life-giving force of the Universal Intelligence that completely fills you up. Open up all of your senses to immerse yourself in this powerful, spiritually charged and potentiated completed action. At this point, say to yourself, "*This action is now completed and fulfilled in the material world. I, with the help of my Higher Self, am now making it happen from within. I am partnering with the Universal Intelligence to create this outcome for my highest good and the good of all concerned.*" Stay in this interior space while repeating and visualizing/feeling your completed action for as long as you feel will be effective. Naturally, the longer you are immersed in this experience, the more deeply you are imprinting this into your consciousness.

Without a doubt, you will find yourself at the right place, at exactly the right time, and with precisely the right person, transforming your inner vision into your everyday reality. When that happens, you will know that your conscious self is not adrift on the ocean without a compass. In fact, by first charting your course and then aligning yourself with the Universal Intelligence, you will quickly come to realize that you have the most accurate GPS available. It is constantly updated every time you set your intention and make it happen from within.

Visualization Technique 2: The star that shines brightly within

This powerful visualization exercise originates from the Tibetan tradition. I learned and have adapted this "dream-changing technique" from teacher and author John Perkins.[12] It is a variation on

Technique 1 (described above) that integrates two of the chakra centers as part of the visualization.

Instead of merging your self-care goal as a completed action within a white circle, visualize sending your completed action into a radiating silver star that is surrounded by darkness. After you visualize this merging taking place, imagine the star coming deep into your forehead, the location of your sixth chakra. This is the chakra that is generally regarded as our energetic center of instant intuitive knowing, spiritual vision and extrasensory perception.

Imagine that the inside of your head is now filled up with powerful and highly reflective crystals, as if transformed into a beautiful crystalline cave. See this star radiating in the very center of your inner crystalline space, embodying the completed action of your self-care goal. Experience the star that contains your completed action exploding three times. Rather than being destroyed, the crystals inside your cranial cave amplify and expand the information that is merged within the star. With each explosion of this highly amplified starburst, feel, sense and affirm its incorporation and imprinting into your mind, nervous system, physical body and all aspects of your being.

After the third explosion, see this star and your completed action sink down into your heart center. Imagine now that your heart center is lined and filled up with powerful and highly reflective crystals that magnify any information that they are exposed to. Again, experience the star that contains your completed action exploding three times. Each time the star and your completed action expand outward, visualize and feel every cell in your body being indelibly imprinted with this information. Know that head and heart are now unified with your intent to actualize your self-care goal. Imagine it already done and let yourself experience your deep conviction that it is now completed.

When you feel ready, allow the star to ascend back up into your head and then back out to its place of origin, radiating your completed action brightly amid the darkness. This time, know that this bright star has been programmed by you to continuously radiate your completed action throughout the universe. Choose a time to do this at least twice a day and wait expectantly for amazing results.

Visualization Technique 3: Contact and communicate with your inner guides

A powerful method for problem solving and generating positive outcomes related to your specific self-care goals is accessing the wise parts of yourself that are often referred to as your inner guides. Unlike the critic figure discussed in Chapter 6, which is a compilation of the many self-devaluing thoughts you have about yourself, interactions with your inner guides allow you to access what seems like an imaginary or magical realm where you can truly know the answer to any question or dilemma.

Though it may sound like a cliché, the solutions to all of your problems reside within you. For many people, this interior knowledge seems well hidden or mysteriously inaccessible. However, you can gain access to these solutions through interacting with your inner guides. To do so, you must be willing to let go of the limiting belief that it is only through your intellect that you can solve your problems. Working with your inner guides is an incredible paradigm-shifting imagery method that will open you up to trusting your intuition, that interior place where you *just know* things to be true.

Inner guides have been referred to throughout history and across a diversity of cultures and traditions. In their various guises, inner guides can be found in the fairy tales and myths of the literature of nearly every society. In the early 1900s, Dr. Carl Jung reintroduced this interior way of working with inner guides, which he called "active imagination," to the Western science of psychology. Jung had his own inner guide, Philemon, with whom he interacted on a regular basis through his active imagination process.

Jung believed his inner guide provided legitimate information that he could trust.

In *The Divine Comedy*, the fourteenth-century preeminent work of Italian literature by Dante Alighieri, Dante's journeys through hell, purgatory and heaven are led by inner guides Virgil and Beatrice. All over the world, indigenous cultures that practice shamanism use percussive drive as a way to create altered states of consciousness so they can access and interact with wise inner guides for divination and healing purposes. Many Christians believe that they have a guardian angel who is with them from birth, often warning them of imminent danger. For many people, inner guides spontaneously emerge in their dreams, providing guidance and sometimes intimations of things to come.

Working with your guides is extremely empowering because you learn to work with your own inner wisdom rather than projecting it onto spiritual teachers, therapists or priests. In other words, *you learn to **own** your knowingness.* Rather than trying to assemble the disparate and often symbolic pieces of confusing dreams, intentionally working with your inner guides expands your consciousness and provides you with answers that emerge from within you.

There are all kinds of ways to intentionally access your inner guides. The method that I outline below is very easy to use. Whether you call it an exercise or a meditation, this approach allows you to cultivate an enduring relationship with one or more inner companions that you grow to trust deeply and can turn to for help when you need answers.

Your first step is to find a location where you won't be distracted. Put a pad of paper and a pen nearby (a digital recorder will also work), since you will want to record your experience after it is over. Get comfortable, close your eyes and allow yourself to relax deeply. Make sure that your body is not distracting you from your task at hand. If you feel fidgety, do some yogic deep breathing by inhaling deeply and holding your breath for seven seconds, followed by an eight-count exhalation. Continue this long deep breathing for three or four minutes. As the tingling subsides, just notice your body letting go of any previous tension.

Now begin thinking about a place that we will call your inner sanctuary. Initially you can think about the many beautiful, tranquil and natural environments that you have visited in your life. It could be a mountain meadow, a resting spot by a waterfall, an open area under a grove of trees in a forest you have hiked, or a place by a river with warming sunshine and a gentle breeze. What matters is that you select a place that you can see vividly and feel good, safe and secure in. When these criteria are met, this interior place becomes your inner sanctuary, a locale you come to visit frequently where you open yourself to connect with your inner guides.

As you spend a few moments orienting yourself to your surroundings, make sure that you're seeing through your eyes and feeling through your body. Your inner reference point is your physical body so that you experience everything in the first person, rather than from a detached position watching yourself. Be as multisensory as you can. Feel the weight of your body as you take a few steps forward. Do you feel a breeze or is the air calm? Is it hot and humid or do you have a sensation of dry warmth on your skin? Next, notice the colors around you. Are you standing on brown composted pine needles and humus in a forest, or a green meadow punctuated by patches of daisies and yellow wildflowers? Try your best to identify and acknowledge the details of your environment. This initial orientation will support your visualization process and activate the circuits in the right side of your brain toward full multisensory immersion.

Once oriented, you have a choice about how to proceed. If you're comfortable taking a more receptive approach, call out your desire for one of your inner guides to approach you where you are standing or sitting. Continue to notice the features of your environment as you continue mentally calling out your request to meet an inner guide. As you wait, maintain an attitude of patience and expectancy. If you prefer taking a more active approach, look around and decide what looks like an interesting direction to begin walking in or an interesting spot you'd like to walk to. At this point, your inner creativity will provide some kind of a device, such as a path or a footbridge. As you move toward your destination, begin calling out your intention to meet one of your guides. Continue to walk around with curiosity, patience and expectancy.

Whichever way you choose to begin your journey, you will soon see in the distance something that is coming toward you. As your inner guide comes closer, you may or may not perceive its form clearly. Sometimes inner guides appear in the form of a glowing light, or a figure with a blurry, indistinct face. If your guide is a figure, is it an animal or a person? Is it male or female?

If you haven't done so already, it's important to suspend your disbelief that you are just making this all up based on stories or movies that you have read or seen in the past. Remember, you are exercising a different part of your brain that you may not have a lot of practice with. Consequently, unless you are used to doing this frequently, you may feel unsure of yourself at first. As well, because you are using the nonrational part of your brain, your experience will be very different from how you normally operate in the outer world of consensus reality. Remember, this is not about thinking! Just don't worry about these concerns and continue on with your inner work. How do you know that this figure is actually one of your true inner guides? *By the feeling that you have* when you're interacting with it. If you feel complete acceptance and even love from this inner guide, it's likely that you've made a solid connection. If you sense any kind of judgment, harshness or negativity emanating from this figure, politely thank it for coming and ask it to leave. Then begin the process over again, asking for a loving, wise, supportive and encouraging inner guide to appear.

Greet this being, introduce yourself, and ask what his or her name is. (For convenience, beginning here I will refer to the guide as "it," since your guide could be a male or female person, an animal or a light.) Accept whatever name comes to you as a first impression. If the guide is a person, ask how old he or she is. Allow yourself to gather impressions about what the figure is like. Is it tall or short? What kind of clothing is it wearing?

Feel free to show your guide around your sanctuary and explore it together. Don't be surprised if your guide points out some things that you hadn't even noticed before. After you have been together for a while and you feel comfortable in its presence, ask your guide if there is something that it would like to tell you, or if there's any advice that it would like to share with you. These are general, open-ended questions, so pay close attention and be receptive. If you have a particular problem that you want help and guidance with, now is a good time to address it. Ask your guide precisely what you've been doing to create the physical symptom or work-related dilemma that you are seeking help with. In other words, ask it to tell you the source of the problem and what you have been doing (or not doing) to perpetuate it. Be curious and proactive—keep the dialogue going by asking as many pertinent questions that you can think of. It's likely that you will receive immediate answers to your queries, but try not to be discouraged if you don't. The answers will come as you learn to trust the process and spend more time with your inner guide.

When you have received all of the information that you think will be helpful, thank your guide and ask if it is willing to share some of its power and vital force with you. If it agrees (as is usually the case), ask if you can gently hold his or her hands (if a person) and look into your guide's eyes to receive what it is willing to transmit to you. Many people feel emotionally overwhelmed at this point and begin to weep from the unexpected sensations and feelings of love coursing through their body. If your guide is a four-legged animal, perhaps you can kneel down and gently hold one or both of its paws while looking into its eyes. In either case, feel the sensations of physical contact with your inner guide through your hands as deeply as you can.

When the experience of being with your guide feels complete and finished, be sure to thank it and ask if there is anything that you can do to honor it as a means of appreciation. Then ask your guide if it is willing to meet you in your sanctuary again. Remember that this needn't be a special occasion. Your guides are available to you anytime you feel the need for support, problem solving assistance or creative inspiration. Whether you choose to meet with any of your guides just once a week or during a daily meditation, they can become reliable inner resources that are always there to support you.

When your exchange is complete, bid your guide good-bye, take a deep breath and slowly return to your normal waking consciousness. Go directly to the pad of paper or recorder you put by your side earlier and write down or record everything that happened. Journeying to one of your inner guides is very much like a dream, so the details of your experience will tend to fade away in a relatively short time.

If you find this exercise helpful emotionally as well as on a practical, problem solving level, consider buying a journal and keeping all of your notes cataloged by date or transferring your MP3 files to a folder on your computer or flash drive.

Overcoming barriers to making your visualizations come true

Once you have established your self-care intention and are reinforcing your new desired beliefs with an ongoing daily visualization process, you mustn't be surprised when resistance to creating this change in your life emerges as doubts and uncertainty. There are a few things that might be at the root of these doubts. Ask yourself the following questions to try to pinpoint what exactly is holding you back from actualizing your self-care goals.

Am I fully committed to making the change?

Am I willing and able to commit the time needed?

Ideally, you should do your creative visualization exercises every day. However, if you are using two or more of the four tools outlined above (creating a vision board and the three numbered techniques), it may be unrealistic to expect yourself to do all four exercises every day. While each of them should be done often—and, of course, the more the better— it's your choice and at your discretion. You may feel that one of the techniques works better for you than the others, and decide to do

> You mustn't be surprised when resistance to creating this change in your life emerges as doubts and uncertainty.

that one every day and the others when you have more time. Or, you may choose to rotate them so you are using them all regularly. Do whatever feels best for you.

Do I truly believe that I can do this?

You may have fallen into the rut of believing that, for one reason or another, it's impossible for you to make any significant changes to your life. Perhaps you feel that you're just trying to survive, dealing with all the responsibilities that are constantly coming at you every day at work and at home. If this is true for you, pause right here and reflect on how committed you are to changing your life. Fundamentally, how much do you really want to live a different life?

Using creative visualization regularly to manifest new realities for yourself is a skill, and like any skill—whether it's playing a musical instrument, dancing the tango or speaking another language—it takes time to learn. This means you must be passionately determined so you can recruit the power of your will and thus command your goal-directed thoughts. When you succeed, your visualizations will ultimately supersede your daily fluctuating emotional feeling states, along with the cravings and aches and pains of your physical body that seem to so often demand your attention.

The natural consequence is that what you constantly direct your attention to or continually think about—in this case, your visualizations—becomes more real to you than anything that you normally orient to in the external world. This is all about your commitment to your self-care goals.

> When a person's focus is so single-minded and mobile that they can transfer all of their attention from their identity onto a thought, action, or object, their frontal lobe will filter out all of the random sensory stimuli in the environment. One hundred percent of their brain's attention becomes centered on the relationship between thought and deed. Essentially, the person's identity is no longer the self with a history; instead, their new identity becomes the thought or the intention they are holding. The mind becomes one with (unified with) whatever they are focusing on.[13]

Reaching this level of commitment to your goals is a kind of self-transcendence, when your mental state generates attentional absorption so focused that, for all practical purposes, you are lost in the moment. This one-pointed state of focused attention has been experienced and described by artists, meditators, athletes and mystics throughout history. If you are willing to practice applying such focused attention in order to transcend the limitations of what you presently believe to be possible (and thus consider the "impossible" as part of your expanding framework of possible outcomes), you will become the creator of your own life. You will be "making it happen from within."

To accomplish this, you must know what you want and it must *feel* more important than anything else in your life at this time. Dr. Andrew Weil's research confirms this:

> Whether the emotion felt as positive or negative seems not to matter; rather it is the intensity of feeling that

gives it power to affect body function. More than negative feelings, apathy may be the major emotional obstacle to spontaneous healing.[14]

Thus, your starting point is your strong desire to realize the explicit self-care goals that you are visualizing regularly, and your undeterred belief that you will succeed in actualizing your goal.

Am I fully congruent with making the change?

You must also be willing and eager to gladly accept this new experience into your life. Are you? The willing acceptance to actually have

> Your starting point is your strong desire to realize the explicit self-care goals that you are visualizing regularly.

what you are seeking is more subtle than many people realize. Whether it's general poor self-esteem or pervasive feelings of shame from growing up in an abusive, dysfunctional family system, not feeling acceptable or okay deep within your core is unfortunately all too common. *If you have the core belief that you deserve all things good, actualizing your goals and intentions will come naturally.*

There really is very little in the way that prevents you from accomplishing whatever you set your mind to. Why shouldn't you have the career that you want and the income that you desire without having to work hours of overtime every day? Why shouldn't you have a mutually respectful, adult loving relationship? And what about all the other successes

> *If you have the core belief that you deserve all things good, actualizing your goals and intentions will come naturally.*

that you secretly wish for but for one reason or another always find excuses for not pursuing?

The underlying reason for not actualizing your goals is generally one or more of those snarly beliefs deeply embedded in your subconscious mind (discussed in Chapter 6) that are generated by your inner critic and your self-limiting beliefs.

Do I have limiting beliefs related to reaching my self-care goals?
Is your present schedule actually interfering with your ability to take care of yourself and be happy? Or is that a limiting belief? Have you always thought of yourself as lazy, comparing yourself to others who are more successful than you are? Might this also be a limiting belief?

Another limiting belief you may have is that you can solve your problems only through the use of your intellect. However, if you are willing to let go of this belief, using visualization techniques and working with your inner guides are incredible paradigm-shifting activities that will open you up to trusting your intuition, that interior place where you *just know* things to be true. As you experience this more consistently, you will truly transform into a human being with extraordinary capacity to make changes in your life.

Is my inner critic holding me back?
An important point to emphasize about creative visualization techniques is that they bypass the logical left-brain thinking process and deliberately engage another dimension of your intelligence. What's more, when your right-brain processing is fully engaged, it's easier to quiet down the critical, doubting part of your mind that may be holding you back from actualizing your ideal life.

But even though you will be able to ignore the critic while you are in a state of inner attentional absorption—that is, while you are focused on visualizing—when you are done the critic can come back to haunt you by sarcastically critiquing and judging your inner work. It may even sabotage your entire process for moving forward to change in the ways that you aspire to. For information on how to confront your inner critic and free yourself from it, see Chapter 6.

By depotentiating the intrusive critic who generates doubts about your abilities to succeed, you will remove many of the barriers that keep you from believing that the change you're working on is possible and likely.

The strategies described in this chapter are not about escapism into dream-like states to temporarily leave your everyday reality for a short-term vacation by altering your consciousness. Addictions tend to serve that purpose, and they are generally self-destructive. On the contrary, getting clear about what you want to change in your life initiates your reflective thinking process to identify what specific changes you need in your life. From here you can begin prioritizing self-care goals, and this is the point at which your imagination starts to fire up.

Creating and holding a specific vision takes commitment and perseverance. Your conscious use of imagery and visualizing is a whole-brain approach to becoming your own creator as you begin to shape your life according to your inner template. I am certain that you have this capacity and can do this.

It has been said that when people are failing in their life they are failing perfectly, because the principles outlined in this chapter are always being used by everyone (albeit frequently not being used consciously). Everyone is always using their imaginative abilities, but many people frequently become fixated on thoughts that make them feel anxious or afraid. As discussed in Chapter 3, the media constantly highlight and reinforce these fears via sensational "news" coverage that perpetuates our feelings of not being safe. This barrage of media information often becomes the barrier to conscious goal setting and becoming a conscious dreamer because people are continually internally rehashing negative images and thoughts that are reinforced by the media. Unfortunately, the underlying laws of thought and manifestation that allow you to change your life in positive ways also apply to changing your life in negative ways. Thus, by focusing on the anxiety- and fear-provoking information

you take in all day, every day, your thoughts are inadvertently changing your life in negative ways. This is why it is so important for you
to be aware of the impact of the Dreaming Media. If you are not
aware of the profound influence that the media have on your inner
reality, the influence is still there—it is just out of your conscious
awareness. *Stay awake* so you don't fall into the enchantment of the
many seductive and persuasive forces vying for your attention wherever you turn. Decide how important it is to achieve your specified
goals, and through consistent practice over time, the choices you
make and the thoughts you focus on will determine the extent of
your success. It has been my intent to provide you with an array
of powerful tools to support your journey for excellent self-care.

As a caregiver or healthcare provider, it's important to acknowledge that all of your problems do have solutions and these solutions
reside inside you. If you can make time to go inside and discover
that interior place where you truly know the answer to any dilemma
that you want to resolve, you will ultimately be more helpful to those
under your charge. If your personal experience confirms that these ideas
and techniques consistently work for
you, your inclination will be to share this wisdom from a place of
rewarding personal experience that becomes your inner knowing.

> It's important to acknowledge that all of your problems do have solutions and these solutions reside inside you.

Questions and Exercises

1. How clear are you about your self-care goals? Write down a
   least three self-care goals that will enhance the quality of your
   life. Engage your imagination and start dreaming about what
   your life will be like when these goals are fully realized.

2. Create a vision board. What self-care goal do you want to
   start with? Let the words and images you put on your vision

board seep into your subconscious mind through daily reinforcement, making it happen from within. Think about it regularly throughout the day, knowing that its realization is now just a matter of time.

3. Are you ready to contact and establish relationships with your inner guides? Promise yourself to make time during the day or in the evening while you still have good mental energy to seek out your guides. Put on some soothing music, get comfortable physically, and write down or record everything you learned from your inner guide when your journey is completed. Know that your inner guides are always available to you for guidance, wisdom and problem solving. Promise to return to your guide soon to discover what kind of power and support it can provide you for your ongoing self-care.

4. As you prepare for sleep, either sitting up or lying down, practice using your multisensory imagination by visualizing certain parts of your day. For example, review a conversation you had with a client or a friend. Remember their tone of voice, the way they moved their body and what clothes they were wearing. Or, imagine yourself achieving one of your high-priority self-care goals. Bring in as much multisensory awareness as you possibly can, remembering that your brain doesn't distinguish between what you have "really seen" versus what you are imagining you are seeing. If you have already created a vision board for this goal, keep it close by so that those outer images start to become mirrored within you with increasing mental clarity. Doing this every night exercises those parts of your brain that are integral for creating and sustaining optimum self-care. Remember that neuroplasticity means that by using repetition you are actually growing different parts of your brain. As these images become more and more imprinted in your neural networks, the vision within

you begins to expand, and the universe outside of you comes ever closer to matching your vision.

5. If you have any kind of chronic physical problem, decide which technique(s) offered in this chapter you will commit to use to resolve and heal the problem. If and when doubts emerge, confront your inner critic and use the technique for correcting psychoenergetic reversal to make sure you are congruent about achieving your success. Work on this daily and expect positive change.

CHAPTER

12

Conclusion

You can give and be a blessing

All the research discussed in Chapter 4 about how powerful our minds truly are is really about the blessings that come to us from helping people and how we as caregivers become blessed in the process. I have provided many examples to help you reassess your ability and willingness to provide profound healing by thinking about yourself differently. My own experience along with this research confirms what you already know—the more you spend time cultivating a daily spiritual or energetic practice, the more you become identified with something greater than yourself. As this happens over time, your identity as a separate individual begins to change as you enlarge your identification and consciousness to include all things in the universe.

Researchers and authors use different metaphors to try to explain their growing awareness of how personal identity must be transformed in order for us to accept that each of us is a healer in our own right. It is an unfortunate myth that only so-called natural-born mystics, healers and holy persons have the ability to heal and create miracles. This mistaken belief marginalizes the rest of us as "average" people who have good intentions but no special gifts to create miraculous healings in others.

So, the first step in considering your ability to bless and heal others *is to believe that you can!* Yet you, like so many people, may think it is presumptuous to see yourself as someone who "blesses" the people you care for if you have not been ordained as a priest or pastor. My contention is that it depends on how you define *blessing*, and whether you consider yourself a person worthy of and willing to bless others.

> The first step in considering your ability to bless and heal others *is to believe that you can!*

At its essence, a blessing occurs when you share your vital force with another so that it touches the heart or the essence of the other person. A blessing needn't be a formalized ritual, since it comes from the heart along with a sense of caring. You can transmit a blessing to another person through your kind words, by offering a reassuring smile, by listening patiently and attentively, or by giving the person a warm embrace. As we have seen, you can even send someone a blessing when you aren't physically together, by using the power of distant prayer and visualization.

> A blessing occurs when you share your vital force with another so that it touches the heart or the essence of the other person.

If the person you are with feels safe and supported by you, a blessing space spontaneously emerges. When this happens, the chi that is transmitted through your presence is felt by the other in a restorative and healing way. According to David Spangler,

> The presence that we can share in the midst of a blessing is one of profound interconnectedness, wholeness, and flow in which there are no obstructions to the manifestation of a oneness within us and between us. I think of this presence as the unobstructed world of spirit. A blessing is an invitation from one person to another to enter into and share this world. It is the opening of a door so we can enter this world together.[1]

Thus, what may appear to be an ordinary visit with someone can become something quite exceptional, since an integral part of the blessing process between you and the other person is your connection to the Sacred.

You must feel connected to Spirit

Some helpers and caregivers are meditators, while others are Reiki practitioners, qigong practitioners or devoted Christians reading scripture as their source of spiritual connection. Your source of inspiration and connection to the Sacred is a completely individual matter. *The key element is that you feel that connection.*

There are many ways in which we can continually strengthen our connection to Source, which also replenishes us so that our vital force remains strong and supportive of all the tasks we choose to take on every day. An ongoing spiritual or energetic practice not only reaffirms our commitment to our well-being and health, but validates our connection to the Greater Mind. This experience confirms that we are not in this alone. Individuals who are willing to make this daily commitment, to live more fully in alignment with Source, are consciously more connected to the nonlocal part of themselves that will energetically transmit that connection to Source to others through their presence. One might say that these individuals have a greater readiness for and access to spiritual realities that can be brought forth as a way to bless others. This kind of daily practice, however you choose to create it for yourself, is self-sustaining and self-nurturing. It will provide you with a deepening sense of how you are blessed with an increasing experience of love and gratitude for the people and situations in your life without undue effort on your part.

Those of us who feel an ongoing connection to the Sacred have at least one characteristic in common—we are all fully present in our physical body. This is what allows us to feel the powerful connection between the Sacred and our heart. The vast majority of caregivers and helpers are naturally deeply empathic, and we already feel so much through our bodies because our emotions are body centered.

If you are dissociated or out of your body, you are undoubtedly cut off from your feelings. In fact, one of our unconscious adaptive responses after having an overwhelming life experience, shock or trauma is to vacate our body in order to cope with the intense emotional aftermath. However, as explained in Chapter 10, you can let go of lingering traumatic residue through energy-based therapies such as Dynamic Energetic Healing®, which includes EFT. You will then be available to feel the joy and the entire spectrum of shifting emotions that accompany your daily interpersonal encounters, and thus confirm for yourself your aliveness in connection to Source and to the person you are with. By learning to stay fully present in your physical body, you allow yourself the experience of vulnerability that comes with letting go of fear and control. You then experience that larger sense of yourself beyond the skin barrier of your physical body and your sense of separateness by risking that connection of relatedness with another. Learning to stay in your physical body while overcoming the inherent vulnerability of your physicality allows you to open yourself up to the force of love that passes between two people. Eventually, this becomes an expression of feeling at home in your body.

While it may seem paradoxical to expand your consciousness to include all things in the universe while at the same time remaining fully present in your own body, I am reminded of a Zen saying: "Before enlightenment, chop wood carry water; after enlightenment, chop wood carry water." Whatever we may imagine enlightenment is, we are still bound to carry on our daily tasks and try to be the best that we can be and fully participate in the world. Staying present to our experience is staying connected to our bodies and thus all of our feelings. From this follows a life lived in deepening authenticity.

The more you are able to live increasingly connected to your experience of Source, the more your life will be blessed, enabling you to share these blessings with others. As David Spangler has written,

> A blessing is much more than just an act. It is an affirmation of our interconnectedness; it is the creation of an opportunity for the power of that connectedness to pour through into our lives and the lives of others. So in practicing the art of blessing, we are really practicing being connected.[2]

If blessing is something that comes from the heart, and from being present with another with deep empathic concern, perhaps caregivers can learn to be the blessing to transform the entire helping process for themselves and the people they help. Caregivers can use the power of their growing connection to Source as well as their focused intention to actually create a greater potential for healing to occur in others. I can't think of a better way to express self-care, stay connected to your body and allow the spiritual power from Source to flow in you and through you freely as you exchange this flow of life force with another.

> The more you are able to live increasingly connected to your experience of Source, the more your life will be blessed, enabling you to share these blessings with others.

I don't believe you need to study esoteric spiritual practices in order for this to happen. To the degree that you are happy and feeling joy within yourself, your energy field and the light and information within it will emanate this and thus communicate energetically all that you are, informing your client with no effort on your part. *Thus, you become the blesser and the blessing.*

As you open yourself to be blessed daily by Spirit through a simple direction of your will, you share blessings with others. As you do this more and more, self-care no longer becomes an ongoing issue. As the great Persian poet Rumi has written, "Reason has no way to its love. Only love opens that secret. If you want to be more alive, love is the truest health."[3]

Amplify your power to bless

While I was connected to one of my inner guides, the following meditation unfolded in my awareness. It gives you a way to focus your attention to your heart field, which enables the emotional frequencies of love, gratitude and unity to be more present in your life wherever you are. This meditation will help you to be both the blesser and the blessing.

Gather up a sheet of paper and some colored pencils. Write the words *love, gratitude* and *unity* in the middle of the paper and put a circle around them. You are now going to create a mind map by writing down the associations to these words that are personally meaningful to you. Using whichever colors feel right to you, draw lines from the words *love, gratitude* and *unity* to your various associations, draw bubbles around each associated word, and then color in the bubbles. Soon, your page may resemble a paisley art work. As you're doing this, feel into your experience when you think of *love, gratitude* and *unity*, and remember specific experiences that elicit those special feelings. Really notice the shapes that emerge as your mind map expands, so that the image of your map seeps into your subconscious. When your map is completed, put it aside for now.

The next step is to acquire a small quartz crystal. To make sure that no one else's energetic influence is in the crystal, you need to cleanse the crystal before using it. You can either place it under cold running water for a minute or so, or smudge it with some burning sage.

When you have prepared your crystal, retrieve your mind map and review it carefully again. When you feel you are done with your review, place your crystal in the middle of your mind map and crumple the paper around the crystal. While holding the crumpled map in your hand, place it against your heart

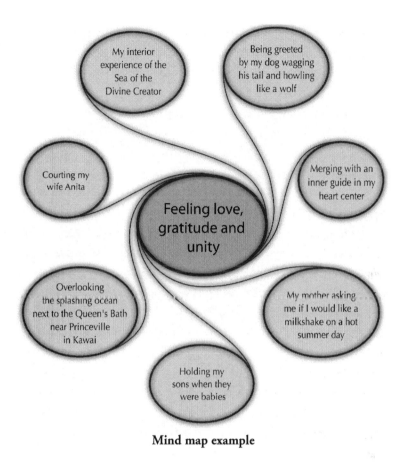

Mind map example

center in the middle of your chest. As you allow your breathing to become long and deep, imagine that you're stoking the fire of the emotional frequencies of *love, gratitude* and *unity* now being absorbed into the crystal. Know that all the associations (the information) that you generated while creating your mind map are being absorbed into this small quartz crystal. Go over in your mind as many of the associations as you can recall. Spend as much time doing this as feels right to you.

This ancient crystal programming technique is powered by the confluence of the loving frequency signatures of the words and colored bubbles on your mind map, which are then amplified as you charge your heart chakra with the chi running through your breath. This deliberate programming process enables the emotional frequencies of *love, gratitude* and *unity* to emanate very powerfully from your heart field. The piezoelectric effect of the crystal (the fact that it receives, stores and transmits electromagnetic energy) will now be constantly positively influencing your thoughts and energy field by radiating these frequencies, much like a satellite transmits its information to its receiver.

When you feel finished, take the crystal out of your mind map and keep it with you at all times—perhaps as a pendant around your neck, or in your pocket. Uncrumple your mind map, take one last look at it, and then throw it away. The information from your map is now energetically programmed into your crystal. Make an effort to place that crystal against your heart center at least once a day as you breathe into and charge your heart center— the seat of compassion—knowing that this breathing meditation process will continually amplify, intensify and charge the crystal that is with you all the time. Pay attention to what you notice over the next three to four weeks as you continue with this daily meditation. While some people might consider this to be a placebo to effect change, let me assure you that your active intentional engagement with your crystal and your heart field will be powerfully and empirically validated as your very presence becomes a blessing.

As we have seen, burnout, compassion fatigue and vicarious trauma can become liabilities and burdens that wear down caregivers over time. But being in a profession or situation in which you are helping someone is a gift and a blessing. This is because of the exquisite nature of the energetic and emotional exchange that happens between people. Yet, no matter how sincere our intentions are

> No matter how sincere our intentions are to help others, we ourselves need help in order to maintain our vital force.

to help others, we ourselves need help in order to maintain our vital force and come back another day to be present for others who have been traumatized, abused or marginalized.

Go on personal retreat

Throughout this book, I have stressed the importance of various self-care strategies, including taking breaks, establishing firm energetic boundaries, and using EFT tapping. In addition to these approaches, making time in your very busy schedule to go on personal retreat is an absolutely essential self-care strategy that every helper or caregiver will benefit from.

It matters little what category of personal retreat you choose. It might be

- spending time alone at a Christian monastery quietly reading, walking and praying
- participating in a Buddhist Vipassana silent meditation retreat for a weekend or a week
- treating yourself to a weekend at a spa
- camping out and fly-fishing or hiking
- taking a weekend workshop in watercolor painting
- learning and practicing shamanic journeywork with a group of people in a week-long workshop

Being on personal retreat gives you the opportunity to unwind your mind and let go of all the preoccupations and ongoing responsibilities that create stress in your life.

Essentially, personal retreat gives you the opportunity to fill yourself up and reconnect to the home frequency of your soul (see Chapter 5 for more information on the concept of home frequency). Additionally, by going on retreat you are doing something

> Personal retreat gives you the opportunity to fill yourself up and reconnect to the home frequency of your soul.

just for you, and providing yourself with time and space in which to reevaluate your daily life. It's the perfect time to reassess and revise agreements you've made with yourself about what you are willing to commit in support of your ongoing personal growth, self-care and spiritual development.

I make the effort to go on a least one meaningful personal retreat every year, and several times have gone to Abadiânia, Brazil, to experience the healing powers of John of God.

John of God

Medium João Teixeira de Faria, also known as John of God, is a world-renowned healer. His guides work through him to provide miraculous healings to the hundreds of people who gather at his healing center, The Casa de Dom Inácio de Loyola, every Wednesday, Thursday and Friday. He is affiliated with the Brazilian spiritist tradition, which is an interesting synthesis of Roman Catholicism and indigenous Brazilian practices.[4]

People who line up to see John of God must traverse three meditation rooms in the process of receiving direction and guidance from the compassionate energies and guides that come through him. Typically, he directs people into a room for focused healing of the problems they are seeking his help with, or into one of three meditation or "current rooms." These current rooms support and maintain the flow of heart-centered spiritual energy that enables the transformative healing forces to come through John of God to do their healing work. As people in the current rooms meditate by asking for the divine energy of universal love to flow through them, a kind of spiritual battery is created. Through this battery, the meditators are nourished by the spiritual energy that is continually renewed and amplified by all the people in the three meditation rooms.

This is a wonderful example of collaboration, for as you are sitting and meditating, opening your heart for the loving energy of the divine to come through you to support those in the focused healing room, you and all the other meditators are being filled up with light and love, and being healed by the compassionate energies and guides at the Casa. This is a fantastic example of group coherence (see Chapter 4), as hundreds of people are all intensely meditating and praying from their heart, creating an energetic field of progressively increasing compassion for everyone who is asking for help.

For five years prior to my first trip to John of God in April of 2003, I had a condition that is often called adrenal exhaustion. I was chronically fatigued on weekends, and felt that my vital energy was depleted—I didn't feel "filled up."

During that five-year period, I found that although acupuncture and traditional Chinese herbs alleviated this pattern of exhaustion by about 70 percent, I was unable to snap back to my previously normal physical energy levels. After reading about John of God, I decided to go on a two-week personal retreat to experience this new healing approach.

When I returned to my acupuncturist after that 2003 retreat with John of God, she felt my pulses and told me that I no longer needed to see her. She said that my mysterious chronic exhaustion was cured. Since then, I have never regressed to that chronic state of exhaustion and my overall energy has been good. In fact, I am able to sustain vigorous cardiovascular exercise regularly during my workweek, something I was unable to do previously.

Since that initial trip in 2003, I have visited John of God a number of times. It is often the case that when I finally get to Abadiânia (a trip that lasts for twenty-three hours) and start adjusting to the slower, less complicated pace of life there, I begin to realize how I really need to rest and restore myself. I have created a lifestyle that is intensely busy, that is fraught with responsibility and activity, and that consumes my daily life. In fact, being so busy with the demands and responsibilities of work and family life frequently precludes me from following my body's needs to rest deeply when tired.

When I'm at the Casa, I realize that my normal approach is to push through any feelings of tiredness in order to attend to the next demand on my schedule, which starts early in the morning and continues late into the evening. I rarely realize how tired I truly am until I am away on personal retreat. It is then that I can finally surrender to the deep tiredness that my body has accumulated over time and spend days just resting, allowing my stores of chi to become replenished.

> I rarely realize how tired I truly am until I am away on personal retreat.

This is always to my great surprise, since I no longer suffer from exhaustion. Upon reflection, I don't consider myself obsessive— I see myself as just another casualty of a strong work ethic and the cultural zeitgeist of twenty-first century America.

Prior to my November 2008 trip to see John of God, I would occasionally muscle test myself on a scale from one to one hundred—with one hundred being the highest degree possible of vital energy circulating throughout my nervous system—and receive a readout from 78 to 98. At the end of my first week in Abadiânia, I was stunned to discover that I was off the chart—my muscle testing readout was 127 relative to the degree of chi circulating in and through my adrenals! Throughout the rest of my stay, my numbers registered between 120 and 127.

When it was time to leave Abadiânia after my two-week retreat in 2008, I felt filled up (with vital force) and complete. I gauged my experience of being filled up by my subjective feeling state. I felt whole, rested, happy and balanced when I left the Casa.

Two weeks after I returned home, I continued to be astounded that my muscle testing registered between 116 and 124. As I write this now in 2011, I regularly come in at 250 to 450! This is extraordinary to me because it indicates that something profound has changed within my core, and that so far I have maintained that new baseline for my energetic integrity. My ongoing physical energy, stamina and overall vitality reflect this.

Staying filled up

I journey to my inner guides (see Chapter 11) regularly as one important aspect of my ongoing spiritual practice. My first two journeys subsequent to my return from Abadiânia in 2008 were revealing and clarifying.

In my first journey to a long-time inner teacher, I was told that the central lesson during my recent personal retreat was all about gathering and storing the powerful spiritual energy that I absorbed while in the meditation or current room sessions at the Casa. This inner teacher told me that I was truly filled up with spiritual power and that it is my task to keep it, maintain it and contain it. I was told not to give my vital force away because that would dissipate my supply, which was keeping all of my physical systems operating at peak efficiency. *I was told that by accumulating and containing this vital force, my very presence energetically would be sufficient to support others in a healing manner.* I understood that this spiritual power in me was so highly charged with vital force that I was now energetically radiating it to clients through my presence.

In other words, I shouldn't exercise my ego and *try too hard* to give of myself to others as a therapist and healer. Though this was a new experiential awareness for me, I was reminded that this is a guiding principle of qigong practice and philosophy. As discussed in Chapter 9, this philosophy focuses on the orientation of just "being" and orienting from my heart instead of doing (or overdoing). Thus, it is now my charge to gather, store and circulate chi rather than naively giving it away from a place of misunderstood compassion. This has a lot to do with the principles of blessing and how many caregivers fall into the energy-depleting orientation of co-dependence (discussed in Chapter 7). This issue is central to caregivers and helpers, who often overextend themselves to the point of emotional and physical burnout.

I would never have experienced these benefits or been given these insights had I not chosen to make personal retreat an essential part of my ongoing self-care. Though there will always appear to be barriers (and thus rationalized "good reasons" or excuses) that prevent you from taking time away from family and work responsibilities, you must decide that it is an absolute priority for your health and well-being to get away and renew yourself in the retreat setting of your choice. While there may be some initial resistance to leave your familiar surroundings in order to "selfishly" do something just for you, reconnecting to your true self will yield ongoing dividends.

> Reconnecting to your true self will yield ongoing dividends.

Final thoughts

While this book is replete with strategies to help you to maintain essential self-care while assisting others, there are a few guiding principles that I want to reiterate for you. These are brief statements that will help you remember what to emphasize as broad themes. Referring to these often will help you enormously to maintain your health and well-being as a high-intensity relater.

Of course, it is important to focus your attention on one thing at a time, reviewing each new concept from each chapter in small portions as you create your own self-care journal. The questions and exercises at the end of each chapter are intended to be part of an ongoing journal so you can keep track of the positive changes as you implement the ideas and strategies that inspire you the most. Start with one theme or big idea and stay with it for at least one week. Don't get trapped into thinking that you must make three or four changes all at once—you will probably become overwhelmed. Think of your self-care as being *the* most important value that everything else in your life depends on.

> Don't get trapped into thinking that you must make three or four changes all at once.

These last questions and exercises are meant as reminders. Consider each one as a weekly meditation to keep coming back to as a way to train your consciousness to pay attention to the particular guiding principle that you are integrating more deeply every day.

1. What do you want for yourself? Be explicit. If you have a number of self-care goals, write them all down. Change them when necessary as your deep inner knowing directs you to. Keep the number manageable. Stay with it until you know absolutely. This is *so* important!

> **What do you want for yourself?**

2. Protect yourself from being violated by other people, even those who you are assisting. Become self-referential. Acknowledge your sensitivity—physically, energetically and emotionally. Observe and study yourself in relationship to your clients, spouse, family members and friends. Notice when you become split and lose or give away a part of yourself to avoid disagreement or conflict. Notice when you feel whole. Make journal entries of when you experience each state. Speak out more frequently about how other peoples' actions affect you (in a nonjudgmental way, of course). Practice saying NO when you really mean it—often. Let people know when their behavior, particularly verbal, violates your limits. Become aware of the critic figure and decide how to stop it in its tracks. Track your own resistance and notice when you emotionally contract during this transition period. Work with a therapist if necessary to get support to establish boundaries and maintain them. Feel yourself becoming empowered and living in full integrity. Make a commitment to stay in your power.

> **Practice saying NO when you really mean it.**

3. Learn to identify energetic vampires and decide what you need to do to maintain your full vitality and preserve your chi so you can avoid becoming depleted and exhausted. Decide what your strategy will be to stay empowered.

4. Practice orienting from your heart field. Discover how intentional you can be and how long you can sustain this. As you find yourself more naturally empathizing with others, notice the unconscious dance of mimicry and rapport occurring. Ask yourself frequently if your empathy is conscious or unconscious. Learn to recognize the difference—your health depends on it.

5. Reflect on the research presented for nonlocal healing and physiological self-coherence. Challenge your present paradigm and consider that orienting from your heart field has a positive energetic influence on all who come into contact with you. Consider the possibility that your presence is a blessing that always benefits those who you are helping. Decide to be the blessing—challenge any limiting beliefs to the contrary.

> Decide to be the blessing—challenge any limiting beliefs to the contrary

6. Develop your own self-rating or self-awareness assessment to identify or somehow measure the degree of your vital force or chi at any given time. Make a list of what you strongly believe, feel and know to be energetically depleting you. Do you work compulsively without significant breaks? Are you constantly tethered to your computer or smart phone? Is the food you eat fast and easy to grab or organic and prepared with care? Journal what you know to be excesses in your life and reflect on what needs to change for greater balance during each day. Track how your overall energy is during the beginning of the

week versus the end of the week, and at the start of the day versus the end of the day. Decide what you need to properly maintain your physical and mental health. Decide that this is important enough to make the time to know.

> Journal what you know to be excesses in your life and reflect on what needs to change for greater balance during each day.

7. As you gain increasing clarity about your self-care goals, observe carefully if psychoenergetic reversal is present. Do you find yourself enthusiastically starting a new self-care practice that you are excited about, only to have it dissipate over the course of weeks? Track this carefully in your self-care journal and determine if the energy psychology strategy of EFT is called for. Determine to succeed.

8. Inquire within to what extent you are aligned with the soul of nature. Spend some dedicated time in nature and pay attention to how much you feel replenished during and after being in a natural environment. Ascertain whether your body keeps directing you to explore this ancient relationship to our earth. Find out if you can determine that the earth really is your original mother that is always available to nurture you.

> Spend some dedicated time in nature and pay attention to how much you feel replenished.

9. Decide how to incorporate your ability to envision your goals. Are you more comfortable with guided visualizations that are accompanied with soothing music and beautifully embellished imagery? Or does the notion of meeting and contacting your inner guides for life direction, guidance and healing appeal to you more? Are you prepared to exercise the discipline to repeatedly visualize a specific self-care or self-healing goal? Since you likely visualize

all the time (although you may not realize it), these suggestions are simply asking you to recruit the powers of your imagination in a focused and structured way to create specific outcomes that you have determined you must have for your well-being and self-care. Once you prove to yourself that you have this inner power, it is easy to add in envisioning the healing and well-being of others as an essential component of your own self-care imagery.

10. Do you schedule personal retreats for yourself as a way to replenish your energies? If this is a new idea to you, think about environments or contexts that you really enjoy being in. Would you prefer a five-day rafting trip in the wilderness, a weekend of beach walking on the coast, a meditative monastic retreat, or perhaps a week-long getaway in London or New York City? The options are infinite. Start dreaming now so you can bring into form a nourishing personal retreat.

High-intensity relaters are drawn to professions that demand emotional engagement. In deeply connecting to others, we feel an attentiveness and aliveness in this interpersonal exchange that is different from what is required in professions that demand more emphasis on technical expertise. The province of caregivers and helpers is the human relationship. The bond that is forged, whether short term or extended, is mysterious and powerful. Perhaps most importantly, it increases the sense of connection for both parties involved. This engagement elicits all the emotions we can feel and don't want to feel—it challenges us as caregivers and helpers to grow beyond our perceived limitations and fears as we learn to reach out to help others in need.

If you chose to isolate yourself and be more like a hermit, you might feel unbothered and relatively safe from intrusion from others, but your personal energy field would likely be self-contained. When you are with another person as a helper, you become expanded and begin to experience an amazing connection to one of the greatest mysteries of life, for aren't we each a living mystery until circumstances draw out qualities from us that are required in the moment?

Helping is fundamental to being human. When someone helps me I feel a deep sense of appreciation, and the experience of a meaningful connection with that person that wasn't there before. I find myself opening up to the energetic and emotional connection that becomes the space between us—it is suddenly *very present* and reassuringly engaging. Any prior sense that I had of aloneness disappears, because I have been recognized and acknowledged at a time of need.

While caregivers and helpers are doing a job within a chosen profession, for most of us it is a calling that is as deeply satisfying as it is demanding. Within this relational space, we learn to open our heart to those who are hurting and grow in compassion. Being fully present with another changes us, because the exchange of vital force creates an interpersonal field of intense energy. Within this field, exchanges of multilevel information are occurring among all participants. This sacred space also helps the person we are with open to their own vulnerability and experience this sacred connection themselves. In this exchange, we gift the other while being gifted ourselves. So long as we consciously exercise ongoing self-care, this link with the other will grow and remain secure. While not without its potential hazards, let us remember all the reasons for entering into this most profound healing space with another. A Persian poet named Hafiz[5] puts it well:

> A Hunting party
> Sometimes has a greater chance

Chapter 12

Of flushing love and God
Out into the open
Than a warrior
All
Alone.

1

About Dynamic Energetic Healing®

There are numerous approaches to counseling, psychotherapy and healing. The method I teach and implement in my private practice is called Dynamic Energetic Healing® (DEH). It is, quite simply, remarkable.

Psychotherapy originated with Sigmund Freud in 1903 with the publication of his book *The Interpretation of Dreams.* Freud called his new healing technique *psychoanalysis.* It is still taught and used today, but because it is expensive and extremely time intensive, it has fallen out of favor with most therapists and clients.

The modern version of Freud's innovation is called talk therapy. Most therapists and counselors use variations of talk therapy and/or cognitive behavioral therapy (CBT). Talk therapy can be very helpful at times, but it has a major limitation—its primary target is your thinking, and its goal is to generate rational insight into your particular problem. It is frequently coupled with pharmaceutical drugs for depression, anxiety and insomnia.

While cognitive behavioral strategies such as "thought stopping" and "cognitive restructuring" are often used, it's hard to *think* yourself out of trauma-related anxiety, depression or post-traumatic stress disorder (PTSD). Like talk therapy, CBT is often coupled with prescription drugs (that can become addictive) to help stabilize your mood. But stabilizing your mood is not the same as healing or resolving your underlying problem. That's where DEH can be very helpful.

Unhealed significant trauma from the past is often responsible for present-day physical and emotional symptoms of distress, including ongoing anxiety, depression, insomnia, substance abuse (including compulsive over-eating) and/or anger control issues. Trauma can be a single incident, such as a traffic accident, the loss of a loved one or a burglary. But trauma can also be something that persists over many years, such as a child being traumatized by growing up in a dysfunctional family in which one or both parents are abusive, alcoholic and/or neglectful. Trauma that persists over months and years often becomes embedded as PTSD (see Chapter 3).

If you have experienced either type of trauma, you may end up with all varieties of ongoing outward symptoms of distress. Internally (and outside of your conscious awareness), dissociated parts of yourself split off from your conscious grasp, taking the traumatic information with them. This is how the underlying roots of the outward symptoms of distress become inaccessible. It's difficult to acknowledge and heal traumatic information that you cannot connect with because it is nonverbal and deeply embedded in feelings and sensations, not thoughts.

When PTSD and other significant traumas remain undetected, they often change your neurochemistry, which results in semi-permanent changes in your mood and behavior. The underlying, unhealed trauma is like an internal satellite that continually broadcasts veiled and painful memories of the trauma that remain under the radar of your conscious awareness. These broadcasts from the unconscious become the persistent outward symptoms of distress that you experience, and the unhealed past traumas generate relationship problems and sabotage important personal goals. If you carry such unresolved trauma, you likely experience significant internal conflicts. At the conscious level, these internal conflicts manifest as confusion and indecision, but they are established and entrenched deep in your unconscious mind. In many cases, these conflicts are the root cause of why you convince yourself (often with illogical reasoning) that you cannot accomplish important goals and realize your personal ambitions.

In other words, as explained in Chapter 6, your inner objections and unconscious limiting beliefs are often responsible for putting the brakes on your motivation. These "brakes" are psychoenergetic reversal, which interferes with your ability to achieve your goals and make positive changes in your life. Your inner objections tend to force you to choose between the two major fears related to making changes in your life: the fear of facing the unknown if you accomplish your desired changes and the fear of continuing to endure the suffering or distress of the present if you don't make the changes.

Dynamic Energetic Healing® is a collaborative process between the client and the therapist/facilitator. Over the course of the therapy, clients gradually learn to trust their own awareness so that they can create and maintain strong and stable interpersonal boundaries (see Chapter 7). Clients also learn how to use an array of powerful tools to gain more control over their own emotional responses and thoughts. These tools can be accessed anytime between the therapy sessions and after the course of therapy is completed. Thus, they become reliable personal resources that can be drawn upon whenever needed.

DEH is an innovative, systematic approach to psychotherapy and counseling that acknowledges, validates and encourages a client's subjective perceptions to be more present by the development of "second attention awareness" (see Chapter 5 in *Dynamic Energetic Healing®*). As a DEH therapist/facilitator, part of my role is to model second attention awareness when I perceive subtle information in the interpersonal field during my interactions with a client. My bringing out what I notice in the moment gives clients permission to trust their own perceptions and to feel safe to bring them out without being judged by their weakening inner critic or by me, the "authority figure" they come to trust.

DEH provides an effective therapeutic context to address relationship issues, blocked emotions, emotional overwhelm and other problems. The treatment process combines energy psychology interventions with manual muscle testing.

Manual muscle testing, which is an important component of applied kinesiology, is used throughout the DEH process. It allows clients to connect directly to their living unconscious through their physical body. Even if clients are consciously confused or somewhat dissociated, it has become evident to me that they can trust their physical body to "tell the truth" (through the muscle testing process), enabling us to access exactly the right information that can identify the underlying source of their presenting issue. Thus, when you participate in DEH sessions, muscle testing gives you and the therapist ongoing feedback from your living unconscious (that is, your physical body). During the process, your inner objections, unconscious limiting beliefs and other significant blocks are gradually identified and released.

This access to the deeply buried originating events allows us to identify and often exhume recent or years-old traumatic residue that reveals itself as one or more of the following:
- negative emotional charge that has remained trapped
- limiting beliefs that provide inaccurate guidance (such as "people can never be trusted") and generate guilt and shame
- overidentification with negative archetypes, such as victim/child or harsh and condemning judge
- blocked or repressed emotions
- compromised and weakened energetic boundaries
- an unconscious desire to die

When trauma has been severe, there is often psychotoxic contamination from an interpersonal encounter that was connected with the trauma. If this contamination is left unattended, it can cause serious ongoing problems for you.

Each of the above aspects of traumatic residue is treated and released during the DEH sessions. Clients leave feeling considerably lighter and excited about how easily they were able to make these changes.

When the originating trauma is released, along with the information it has been unconsciously broadcasting, real and noticeable change happens and profound healing can occur. Your neurochemistry then tends to come back into balance naturally. Once this information (the traumatic residue) is released through the various energy-based strategies and interventions that are used in DEH, it tends to stay released, which enables you to successfully move forward on your chosen therapeutic goals.

Discussion of therapeutic goals and underlying problem states is central to this approach. However, DEH is not conventional talk therapy because it goes beyond the rational intellect to use your physical body's innate connection to your unconscious vault. DEH allows you to easily access and open that vault in a way that is gentle and effective.

Another distinguishing characteristic of DEH is the relative ease and effectiveness with which hidden and unidentified traumas from your past are identified and released. Talk therapy and CBT often take years before you experience lasting positive outcomes. DEH bypasses the seemingly endless hours of talking about and rationally analyzing your outward symptoms. DEH is an evolving reflection of the need to get problems resolved more rapidly in order to keep up with changing times and keep down costs.

Dynamic Energetic Healing® is a synthesis of ancient energy-based modalities with contemporary evidence-based psychological methods to create positive shifts in your thinking, behavior and emotional life. Many people find it to be exactly what they are looking for. For more information about DEH, please visit my website:

www.DynamicEnergeticHealing.com

2

Self-Assessment Checklists for High-Intensity Relaters

The following checklists will help you determine your current level of risk of experiencing secondary trauma, burnout and compassion fatigue. They will also help you to identify the degree of satisfaction you get from helping others. Taking the time to complete these subjective self-assessments will help you identify both the positive and the damaging aspects of your experience being in direct contact with other people in a helping context.

Completing the checklists

- Be as honest as you can about what your present experience is helping others.
- If the answer is *never*, write an **N** next to the question.
- If the answer is *sometimes*, write an **S** next to the question.
- If the answer is *often*, write an **O** next to the question.

For simplicity, the checklists are phrased to apply to professional caregivers and helpers. That is, they refer to *clients* and *co-workers*. But these checklists apply equally well to nonprofessionals who are caring for loved ones at home or in other settings. If you are part of this second group, substitute *loved one* for *client*, and *other family members* or *other helpers* for *co-workers*.

Checklist #1: Your *positive* responses to being a helper

Am I happy and fulfilled?
___ Overall, I am happy and content.
___ My life and my work are satisfying to me.
___ I feel calm and emotionally balanced most of the time.
___ I know I'm a sensitive person, and I'm OK with that.
___ I am happy with the person I have become.
___ Even though my work as a caregiver is very demanding, I'm happy to be helping people who have significant problems.
___ Helping others brings me a lot of personal gratification.
___ Helping others makes me feel good about myself.
___ I intend to be a helper for a long time.

Is my work a positive experience for me?
___ I look forward to helping the people who I take care of.
___ I deeply enjoy my work as a helper or caregiver.
___ I feel connected to other people at work and outside of work.
___ I enjoy interacting with my co-workers.
___ I often feel invigorated and energized after working with the people I help.
___ Some people I help are especially inspiring to me and stimulating to work with.
___ I regularly discover and learn new things from the people I care for.
___ I make sure to keep up-to-date with new therapeutic techniques and other developments in my field.
___ Helping others in pain has made me realize how much compassion I have.
___ I pride myself in being a good helper.

How well am I taking care of myself?
___ I can maintain strong energetic boundaries with my clients.

____ I have regular self-care practices I do that help me stay centered to do my work as a helper or caregiver.

____ I have a good balance between my work and the rest of my life.

____ I can finally say that I don't take work home with me, and I don't think about clients' problems once I leave work.

____ I can keep a positive attitude about my job as a helper or caregiver even though I have to do paperwork too.

Do I have a strong support system?

____ I get enough support from colleagues, friends and family when I'm under a lot of stress.

____ I can depend on my co-workers to help me out when I need support.

____ I am available to help my co-workers when they need it.

____ I have a supportive therapist I can go to when I need to process work-related issues.

____ I have a patient and understanding partner who listens to me when I need to blow off some steam.

Checklist #2: Your *negative* responses to being a helper

How does my work make me feel emotionally and physically?

____ My work as a helper generates stress symptoms in me.

____ I feel overwhelmed by my work as a helper.

____ Being a helper makes me feel weak, tired, and even exhausted.

____ Being a helper makes me feel depressed.

____ Somehow, being a helper or caregiver makes me feel worthless.

____ I lose my temper over little things.

____ At times my anger seems out of control.

____ I work too hard and don't make enough time for myself.

____ I get a feeling of hopelessness when I'm helping others.

____ I feel tense and anxious about helping some people.

____ I feel like a failure or a fraud as a helper.

____ I feel alienated from others.

____ I often feel I should be paid a lot more for all my hard work.

How vulnerable do I feel?

____ I "catch" other people's negative feelings too easily.

____ Setting firm boundaries with people who are suffering is difficult for me.

____ I'm afraid that I might have been "infected" by the residual trauma of those I help.

____ I have to remind myself to be emotionally detached about the well-being of the people I help.

____ It's hard for me to say NO to people who need help and support. I allow people I work with to take advantage of my kind nature.

____ I change the subject with clients when their experience is too awful for me to hear.

____ I avoid certain activities or situations because they make me feel overwhelmed.

____ There are some people I help whose judgmental qualities make me anxious.

Do my circumstances (past and present) make things easier for me, or more difficult?

____ I grew up in a family where verbal and physical abuse was common.

____ I experienced trauma during my childhood.

____ I have experienced trauma in my own adult life.

____ I have "unfinished business" related to specific traumatic experiences from my past that I need to take care of, but I keep avoiding it.

____ I don't have many close friends but would like that in
my life.

____ I have no one to talk to about the stress I'm regularly under.

Are there signs that I'm starting to feel burned out?

____ I have trouble getting to sleep or staying asleep.

____ I startle easily at work and/or at home.

____ I get frustrated having to do the routine tasks in my work as
a helper.

____ While working with abused clients, I feel angry toward the
abuser who hurt my client.

____ I want to avoid helping certain people.

____ I feel in danger working with the people I help.

I perceive that some people I help wish I would just go
away.

____ I feel like I'm just treading water in my life, and that I'm
not achieving my life goals.

____ I have flashbacks associated with those I help.

____ I'm working more for the money than for personal
fulfillment.

____ I find it hard to keep my personal life and my "helper" life
separate.

____ By the end of the week, I feel like I have nothing left to give.

What do your results mean?

When you have completed the questions, follow the steps to com-
pile your results and consider your present situation as a high-
intensity relater:

Number of *often* answers in Checklist #1:   _____

Number of *sometimes* and *never* answers in Checklist #2: _____

Total: _____

If your Total is 38 or more,

• Chances are that you are maintaining your overall health and well-being in spite of working in challenging circumstances. The higher your score is, the closer you are to being a healthy caregiver or helper that exemplifies optimal self-care.

If your Total is less than 38,

• You may be dealing with compassion fatigue or secondary trauma, even if you have not sufficiently acknowledged it before now. I urge you to explore ways to support your self-care sooner rather than later. A very important first step is to ask around for a recommended therapist or counselor with whom you'll feel comfortable discussing these issues. Perhaps your supervisor or family doctor can suggest one.

• Evidently, there are a number of helping or caregiving issues that remain unresolved for you. Perhaps you need to work on establishing better boundaries with those you help. Be honest with yourself about where you are at and acknowledge your feelings.

Note: This measurement tool isn't meant to "diagnose" you or to be the final word on how well you're taking care of yourself right now. Instead, it gives you a general indication of how well or how poorly you are doing as a caregiver or helper. It is worthwhile spending some time reviewing your responses, especially the statements to which you answered 'often'.

• The more you answer 'often' in Checklist #1, the more likely it is that you are managing to take good care of yourself in your interactions as a caregiver or helper.

• The more you answer 'often' in Checklist #2, the more likely it is that you are minimizing or trying to ignore your work-related stressors, and that you may be more at risk than you care to admit.

Burnout and secondary traumatization can creep up on you gradually, and relying on your memory of how you felt four, eight, or twelve months ago will not give you an accurate sense of whether you're sliding toward burnout, holding your own, or getting better at taking care of yourself.

The important thing is to be honest with yourself about your current situation right now and how it is affecting you, both positively and negatively. If you need some help or support, don't be shy or hesitant about asking for it. Do whatever is necessary to maintain your health and well-being because for all that you do for others, you deserve it.

If you would like to download these checklists, go to

www.DynamicEnergeticHealing.com

then click **Order Books** on the main navigation bar.

NOTES

Chapter 1

1. http://www.census.gov/popest/, assessed on April 25, 2012.
2. St. Petersburg Bar Association Magazine, "Compassion Fatigue—Because You Care," assessed February 2007, http://www.lpac.ca/main/articles_bibs/vicarious_bib.aspx, accessed on April 25, 2012.
3. A. Pines and C. Maslach, "Characteristics of Staff Burnout in Mental Health Settings," *Hospital and Community Psychiatry* 29, no. 4 (1978), found in Rothschild and Rand, *Help for the Helper*, 12.
4. L. C. Terr, "Psychic Trauma in Children and Adolescents," *Psychiatric Clinics of North America* 8, no. 4 (1985), found in Rothschild and Rand, *Help for the Helper*, 12.
5. Figley, *Compassion Fatigue.*
6. Brockman, *Dynamic Energetic Healing®.*

Chapter 2

1. *The American Heritage® Dictionary of the English Language*, 4th ed. (New York: Houghton Mifflin, 2006).
2. *The American Heritage® New Dictionary of Cultural Literacy*, 3rd ed. (New York: Houghton Mifflin, 2005).
3. Douglas Harper, *Etymology Dictionary*, accessed February 5, 2012, http://www.etymon line.com. German philosopher Rudolf Lotze coined in Einfühlung ("in-feeling" or "feeling-into") in 1858, based on the Greek word empatheia (passion). The first use of the word *empathy* in English print was in 1903. *Empathize* as a verb was coined in 1924. Note that these dates should be taken as approximate, since a word may have been used in conversation for hundreds of years before it turns up in a manuscript that has survived the centuries.
4. Gardner, *Multiple Intelligences: New Horizons*, 3.
5. Gardner, *Multiple Intelligences: The Theory in Practice*, 9.
6. Howard Gardner and Thomas Hatch, "Educational Implications of the Theory of Multiple Intelligences," *Educational Researcher* 18, no. 8 (1989), quoted in Goleman, *Emotional Intelligence*, 39.
7. Brockman, *Dynamic Energetic Healing®*, 207, 299.
8. Baron and Wagele, *The Enneagram Made Easy.*
9. Aron, *The Highly Sensitive Person*, ix.
10. Aron, *The Highly Sensitive Person*, 7.
11. Aron, *The Highly Sensitive Person*, 8.
12. Orloff, *Positive Energy*, 11.

13. Orloff, *Positive Energy*, 21.
14. Orloff, *Positive Energy*, 22.
15. Orloff, *Positive Energy*, 25.
16. Baron and Wagele, *The Enneagram Made Easy*.

Chapter 3

1. http://www.proactivechange.com/stress/statistics.htm. This information is based on a study done by the American Psychological Association in 2007. Assessed April 25, 2012.
2. Alex Veiga, "US Homes Lost to Foreclosure Up 25% on Year," *USA Today*. September 17, 2010, http://www.usatoday.com/money/topstories/2010-09-16-4155958592 _x.htm.
3. "Home buyers rush to use tax credits," *Statesman Journal* (Salem, Oregon), April 30, 2010, Business section.
4. *Statesman Journal*, March 27, 2011, front page.
5. *Statesman Journal*, March 27, 2011, front page.
6. Brockman, *Dynamic Energetic Healing*®.
7. *The American Heritage*® *Dictionary of the English Language*, 4th ed. (New York: Houghton Mifflin, 2004), accessed February 14, 2004, http://dictionary.reference.com/browse/allopathic.
8. http://nccam.nih.gov/news/camstats/2007/camsurvey_fs1.htm.
9. Michael A. Morton and Mary Morton, *Five Steps to Selecting the Best Alternative Medicine* (New World Library, 1997), accessed December 6, 2011, https://www.healthy.net/scr/Article.aspx?Id=510&xcntr=3. Assessed April 25, 2012.
10. http://www.pbs.org/empires/thegreeks/background/7_p1.html, accessed December 6, 2011.
11. Anand Giridharadas, "In Cellphone, India Reveals an Essence," *The New York Times*, May 7, 2009, accessed February 5, 2012, http://www.nytimes.com/2009/05/08/ world/asia/08iht -letter.html?scp=1&sq=in%20cell%20phone%20india%20 reveals&st=cse.
12. TV-Free America, "How Television Affects Our Lives," *The Peace- worker* (Salem, Oregon), November 30, 2009, accessed February 1, 2012, http://peaceworker.dreamhosters.com/2009/11/how-television -affects-our-lives/.
13. Alicia Ashby, "World of Warcraft Passes 12M Subscribers," *Engage Digital*, October 8, 2010, accessed on February 1, 2012, http://www.engagedigital.com/2010/10/08/ world-of-warcraft-passes -12m-subscribers.

Chapter 4

1. Dossey, *Reinventing Medicine*, 19.
2. Dossey, *Reinventing Medicine*, 24.
3. Dossey, *Prayer Is Good Medicine*, 32.
4. Dossey, *Prayer Is Good Medicine*, 49.
5. Dossey, *Reinventing Medicine*, 37.
6. Dossey, *Reinventing Medicine*, 54.
7. Dossey, *Reinventing Medicine*, 55.
8. Dossey, *Reinventing Medicine*, 49.
9. Brockman, *Dynamic Energetic Healing*®, 73.
10. Dossey, *Reinventing Medicine*, 72.
11. Philip Ball, "The Memory of Water," *nature.com*, accessed February 5, 2012, http://www.nature.com/news/2004/041004/full/news041004 -19.html.
12. Emoto, *Hidden Messages*.
13. Emoto, *Hidden Messages*, 43.
14. Emoto, *Hidden Messages*, xxiv.
15. Emoto, *Hidden Messages*, 90.
16. For example, see Kristopher Setchfield, "Review and Analysis of Dr. Masaru Emoto's Published Work on the Effects of External Stimuli on the Structural Formation of Ice Crystals," December 20, 2005, accessed February 1, 2012, http://www.is-masaru-emoto-for-real.com. Setchfield has this to say about Emoto's research: "While [Emoto] does employ the spirit of the scientific method in his research design, he makes critical mistakes in its rigor. . . . Dr. Emoto's procedure for photographing crystals has no controlled means of ensuring that experimenter's bias is prevented or minimized. . . . Dr. Emoto specifi-cally stated, 'I do not require any blind tests on any samples.' . . . While it is possible that he did, in fact, discover that water has an observable sensitivity to external stimuli such as prayer and words, Dr. Emoto's experimental design and clinical procedures do not prove the claim. A double blind procedure in which a photographer would not know what water sample he or she was photographing would make the claim considerably more credible." Further discussion on the validity of Dr. Emoto's research with water crystals can be found in Diana Rico, "Scientists Investigate Water Memory," *Odewire*, accessed December 8, 2011, http://odewire.com/170441/scientists-investigate -water-memory.html, and in Lionel Milgrom, "Icy Claim That Water Has Memory," *New Scientist*, June 11, 2003, accessed February 1, 2012, http://www.newscientist.com/article/dn3817-icy-claim-that -water-has-memory.html.

17. Rick Jervis, "Directing Flow of Money from BP Spill," *USA Today*, December 6, 2011.
18. Dossey, *Reinventing Medicine*, 83.
19. Hagelin, "The Power of the Collective."
20. Orme-Johnson, et al., "International Peace Project."
21. Hagelin, "The Power of the Collective," 17.
22. Hagelin, "The Power of the Collective," 19.
23. Dossey, *Reinventing Medicine*, 83.
24. Dossey, *Reinventing Medicine*, 112.
25. McTaggart, *The Field*, 103.

Chapter 5

1. Goleman, *Emotional Intelligence*, 97.
2. Rothschild and Rand, *Help for the Helper*, 77.
3. Hatfield, Cacioppo, and Rapson, *Emotional Contagion*.
4. Rothschild and Rand, *Help for the Helper*, 50, 54.
5. Stern, *Interpersonal World*, 30.
6. Brockman, *Dynamic Energetic Healing*®, 53–59.
7. Peirce, *Frequency*, 100, 105.
8. Peirce, *Frequency*, quoted in Bradley, McCraty, and Tomasino, "The Resonant Heart."
9. Bradley, McCraty, and Tomasino, "The Resonant Heart."
10. Bynner, *The Way of Life*, 55.

Chapter 6

1. Dispenza, *Evolve Your Brain*, 43.
2. Dispenza, *Evolve Your Brain*, 43.
3. Dispenza, *Evolve Your Brain*, 449.
4. Callahan and Trubo, *Tapping the Healer Within*, 84.

Chapter 7

1. Brockman, *Dynamic Energetic Healing*®, 33.
2. Brockman, *Dynamic Energetic Healing*®, 139.
3. Schaef, *Co-Dependence*, 44.
4. Schaef, *Co-Dependence*, 58.
5. Orloff, *Positive Energy*, 290.
6. Orloff, *Positive Energy*, 298.
7. Figley, *Treating Compassion Fatigue*, 155.
8. Brockman, *Dynamic Energetic Healing*®, 224.

9. Marcia Bagnall, "What Businesses Can Learn from Steve Jobs," *Statesman Journal*, October 9, 2011, Inside Business section.

Chapter 8

1. Pollan, *In Defense of Food*, 116.
2. Pollan, *In Defense of Food*, 81.
3. Perkins, *Shape Shifting*, 115.
4. Perkins, *Shape Shifting*, 116.
5. Buhner, *Lost Language of Plants*, 37–38.
6. Buhner, *Lost Language of Plants*, 228.
7. Buhner, *Lost Language of Plants*, 227.
8. Buhner, *Lost Language of Plants*, 132.
9. http://www.nelsonsnaturalworld.com/en-gb/uk/our-brands/bach originalflowerremedies/welcome/, accessed February 5, 2012.
10. Edward Bach, quoted in Bach and Wheeler, *The Bach Flower Remedies*, 47.
11. See pages 157–165.
12. Edward Bach, quoted in Bach and Wheeler, *The Bach Flower Remedies*, 62.
13. See page 199.
14. Kaminski and Katz, *Flower Essence Repertory*, 27.

Chapter 9

1. Jahnke, *The Healing Promise of Qi*, 25.
2. Ener-G-Polari-T, "Testing Results," http://www.energpolarit.com /category.aspx?cid=230.
3. See Lisa James, "Good Hydration," June 17, 2004, accessed June 14, 2009, http://vitanetonline.com/forums/1/Thread/317.
4. http://www.mercola.com/article/water.htm.
5. Andrew Weil, response to "Can sleep deprivation make you sick?" http://www.drweil.com/drw/u/QAA366281/sleep-deprivation, May 19, 2006.
6. Brockman, *Dynamic Energetic Healing*®.
7. http://en.wikipedia.org/wiki/Wu_wei
8. For more information on this type of meditation, see Sakyong Mipham's Turning the Mind Into an Ally.
9. Jahnke, *The Healing Promise of Qi*, 114.

Chapter 10

1. Brockman, *Dynamic Energetic Healing*®, 91.
2. David Feinstein, "Energy Psychology: A Review of the Preliminary Evidence," *Psychotherapy Theory, Research, Practice*, Training 45, no. 2

(2008), http://www.innersource.net/ep/articlespublished
/researchoverview.html.
3. Eden and Feinstein, *Energy Medicine*, 63–69.
4. Eden and Feinstein, *Energy Medicine*, 97.
5. Hass, *EFT*, 32.
6. Joaquin Andrade and David Feinstein, "Energy Psychology: Theory, Indications, Evidence," in Feinstein, *Energy Psychology Interactive*, 199–214.

Chapter 11

1. Christina 123, "Cab Drivers Have an Enlarged Hippocampus: Scientific Fact!" *NowPublic*, September 11, 2008, accessed February 1, 2012, http://www.nowpublic.com/health/cab-drivers-have enlarged -hippocampus-scientific-fact.
2. Dispenza, *Evolve Your Brain*, 49.
3. Dispenza, *Evolve Your Brain*, 409.
4. Newberg and Waldman, *How God Changes Your Brain*.
5. Quoted in Denning and Phillips, *Practical Guide*, 128.
6. Dispenza, *Evolve Your Brain*, 475.
7. Ostrander, Schroeder, and Ostrander, *Super-Learning*.
8. De Mille, *Put Your Mother on the Ceiling*.
9. Naparstek, *Invisible Heroes*.
10. Naparstek, *Invisible Heroes*, 203.
11. This visualization is an adaptation of the "Charging Technique" in Denning and Phillips, *Practical Guide*, 96.
12. Perkins, *Shape Shifting*, 89–90.
13. Dispenza, *Evolve Your Brain*, 371.
14. Weil, *Spontaneous Healing*, 201.

Chapter 12

1. Spangler, *Blessing*, 61.
2. Spangler, *Blessing*, 17.
3. Coleman Barks, trans., *Rumi: The Book of Love: Poems of Ecstasy and Longing* (New York: HarperSanFrancisco, 2003), 117.
4. For more information on the Brazilian spiritist tradition, see Allan Kardec, *The Spirits' Book*.
5. *The Gift: Poems by Hafiz, The Great Sufi Master*, Daniel Ladinsky, trans. (New York: Penguin, 1999), 26.

BIBLIOGRAPHY

Aron, Elaine N. *The Highly Sensitive Person: How to Thrive When the World Overwhelms You.* New York: Broadway Books, 1996.

Bach, Edward, and F.J. Wheeler. *The Bach Flower Remedies* (includes *Heal Thyself, The Twelve Healers,* and *The Bach Remedies Repertory*). New Canaan, CT: Keats, 1997.

Baron, Renee, and Elizabeth Wagele. *The Enneagram Made Easy: Discover the 9 Types of People.* San Francisco: Harper, 1994.

Bradley, R.T., R. McCraty, and D. Tomasino. "The Resonant Heart." Shift 5 (2005), accessed February 1, 2012, http://www.noetic.org/library/magazines/shift-issue-5/2/.

Bradshaw, John. *Healing the Shame That Binds You.* 2nd ed. Deerfield Beach, FL: Health Communications Inc., 2005.

Brockman, Howard. *Dynamic Energetic Healing®: Integrating Core Shamanic Practices with Energy Psychology Applications and Processwork Principles.* Salem, OR: Columbia Press, 2006.

Bry, Adelaide, and Marjorie Bair. *Visualization: Directing the Movies of Your Mind.* New York: Barnes and Noble Books, 1978.

Buhner, Stephen Harrod. *The Lost Language of Plants: The Ecological Importance of Plant Medicines to Life on Earth.* White River Junction, VT: Chelsea Green, 2002.

Bynner, Witter, trans. *The Way of Life According to Lao Tzu.* New York: Capricorn Books, 1962.

Callahan, Roger, and Richard Trubo. *Tapping the Healer Within: Using Thought-Field Therapy to Instantly Conquer Your Fears, Anxieties, and Emotional Distress.* New York: McGraw-Hill, 2002.

Cumming, Heather, and Karen Leffler. *John of God: The Brazilian Healer Who's Touched the Lives of Millions.* Hillsboro, OR: Beyond Words, 2007.

De Mille, Richard. *Put Your Mother on the Ceiling: Children's Imagination Games.* Gouldsboro, ME: The Gestalt Journal Press, 1955.

Denning, Melita, and Osborne Phillips. *Practical Guide to Creative Visualization: Manifest Your Desires.* St. Paul, MN: Llewllyn, 1980.

Dispenza, Joe. *Evolve Your Brain: The Science of Changing Your Mind.* Deerfield Beach, FL: Health Communications Inc., 2007.

Dossey, Larry. *Prayer Is Good Medicine.* New York: HarperSanFrancisco, 1996.

———. *Reinventing Medicine: Beyond Mind-Body to a New Era of Healing.* New York: HarperSanFrancisco, 1999.

Eden, Donna, and David Feinstein. *Energy Medicine: Balance Your Body's Energies for Optimum Health, Joy, and Vitality.* New York: Jeremy P. Tarcher/Putnam, 1998.

Emoto, Masaru. *The Hidden Messages in Water.* Translated by D.A. Thayne. Hillsboro, OR: Beyond Words, 2004.

Feinstein, David. "Energy Psychology: A Review of the Preliminary Evidence." *Psychotherapy: Theory, Research, Practice, Training* 45, no. 2 (2008): 199–213, http://www.innersource.net/ep/articlespublished.

———. *Energy Psychology Interactive: An Integrated Book and CD Program for Learning the Fundamentals of Energy Psychology.* Ashland, OR: Innersource, 1994.

Figley, Charles R., ed. *Compassion Fatigue: Coping with Secondary Traumatic Stress Disorder in Those Who Treat the Traumatized.* London: Brunner-Routledge, 1995.

———. *Treating Compassion Fatigue.* New York: Routledge Taylor & Francis, 2002.

Gallo, Fred P., *Energy Psychology: Explorations at the Interface of Energy, Cognition, Behavior, and Health.* Boca Raton, Florida: CRC Press LLC, 1999.

Gardner, Howard. *Frames of Mind: The Theory of Multiple Intelligences.* New York: Basic Books, 1983.

———. *Intelligence Reframed: Multiple Intelligences for the 21st Century.* New York: Basic Books, 1999.

———. *Multiple Intelligences: The Theory in Practice.* New York: Basic Books, 1993.

————. *Multiple Intelligences: New Horizons.* New York: Basic Books, 2006.

Gawain, Shakti. *Creative Visualization: Use the Power of Your Imagination to Create What You Want in Your Life.* Novato, CA: Nataraj Publishing, 1978.

Gladwell, Malcolm. *Blink: The Power of Thinking Without Thinking.* London, UK: Penguin Books, 2005.

Goleman, Daniel. *Emotional Intelligence: Why It Can Matter More Than IQ.* New York: Bantam Books, 1995.

Hagelin, John. "The Power of the Collective." *Shift* 15 (2007), http://www.noetic.org/ library/publication-articles/power-collective/.

Hass, Rue Anne. *EFT: Emotional Freedom Techniques for the Highly Sensitive Temperament.* Fulton, CA: Energy Psychology Press, 2009.

Hatfield, Elaine, John T. Cacioppo, and Richard L. Rapson. *Emotional Contagion: Studies in Emotion and Social Interaction.* Cambridge, UK: Cambridge University Press, 1993.

Jahnke, Roger. *The Healing Promise of Qi: Creating Extraordinary Wellness through Qigong and Tai Chi.* Chicago: Contemporary Books, 2002.

Kaminski, Patricia, and Richard Katz. *Flower Essence Repertory: A Comprehensive Guide to North American and English Flower Essences for Emotional and Spiritual Well-Being.* Nevada City, CA: The Flower Essence Society, 1986.

Kardec, Allan. *The Spirits' Book.* Translated by Anna Blackwell. Conselho Espirita Internacional (International Spiritist Council), 2008.

Katherine, Anne. *Where to Draw the Line: How to Set Healthy Boundaries Every Day.* New York: Simon & Schuster, 2000.

Laney, Marti Olsen. *The Introvert Advantage: How to Thrive in an Extrovert World.* New York: Workman, 2002.

Langshur, Eric, Sharon Langshur, and Mary Beth Sammons. *We Carry Each Other: Getting through Life's Toughest Times.* San Francisco: Conari Press, 2007.

McTaggart, Lynne. *The Field: The Quest for the Secret Force of the Universe.* New York: HarperCollins, 2002.

Mipham, Sakyong. *Turning the Mind Into an Ally.* New York: Riverhead Books, 2003.

Naparstek, Belleruth. *Invisible Heroes: Survivors of Trauma and How They Heal.* New York: Bantam Dell, 2004.

Newberg, Andrew, and Mark Robert Waldman. *How God Changes Your Brain: Breakthrough Findings from a Leading Neuroscientist.* New York: Ballantine Books, 2009.

Orloff, Judith. *Positive Energy: 10 Extraordinary Prescriptions for Transforming Fatigue, Stress and Fear into Vibrance, Strength and Love.* New York: Three Rivers Press, 2004.

Orme-Johnson, D.W., C.N. Alexander, J.L. Davies, H.M. Chandler, and W.E. Larimore. "International Peace Project in the Middle East: The Effects of the Maharishi Technology of the Unified Field." *Journal of Conflict Resolution* 32 (1988): 776–812.

Osmont, Kelly, and Marilyn McFarlane. *Parting Is Not Goodbye... Coping with Grief in Creative, Healthy Ways.* Portland, OR: Nobility Press, 1986.

Ostrander, Sheila, Lynn Schroeder, and Nancy Ostrander. *Super-Learning.* New York: Laurel, 1982.

Peirce, Penney. Frequency: *The Power of Personal Vibration.* Hillsboro, OR: Beyond Words, 2009.

Perkins, John. *Hoodwinked.* New York: Broadway Books, 2009.

———. *Shape Shifting: Techniques for Global and Personal Transformation.* Rochester, VT: Destiny Books, 1997.

Pollan, Michael. *In Defense of Food: An Eater's Manifesto.* New York: Penguin Books, 2008.

Poole, Judith. *More Than Meets the Eye: Energy.* Watertown, MA: Pooled Resources, 1999.

Robertson, Ian. *Opening the Mind's Eye: How Images and Language Teach Us How to See.* New York: St. Martin's, 2002.

Rothschild, Babette, and Marjorie Rand. *Help for the Helper: Self-Care Strategies for Managing Burnout and Stress.* New York: Norton & Company, 2006.

Schaef, Anne Wilson. *Co-Dependence: Misunderstood—Mistreated.* San Francisco: Harper & Row, 1986.

Schwartz, Gary, and Linda Russek. *The Living Energy Universe: A Fundamental Discovery that Transforms Science & Medicine.* Charlottesville, VA: Hampton Roads, 1999.

Skovholt, Thomas M. The *Resilient Practitioner: Burnout Prevention and Self-Care Strategies for Counselors, Therapists, Teachers, and Health Professionals.* Boston, MA: Allyn & Bacon, 2001.

Sobel, Eliezer. *The 99th Monkey: A Spiritual Journalist's Misadventures with Gurus, Messiahs, Sex, Psychedelics, and Other Consciousness-Raising Experiments.* Santa Monica, CA: Santa Monica Press, 2008.

Spangler, David. *Blessing: The Art and the Practice.* New York: Riverhead Books, 2001.

Steinbrecher, Edwin C. *The Inner Guide Meditation: A Spiritual Technology for the 21st Century.* New Beach, ME: Samuel Weiser, 1988.

Stern, Daniel N. *The Interpersonal World of the Infant.* New York: Basic Books, 1987.

Weil, Andrew. *Spontaneous Healing: How to Discover and Enhance Your Body's Natural Ability to Maintain and Heal Itself.* New York: Alfred A. Knopf, 1995.

Wright, Machaelle Small. *Flower Essences: Reordering Our Understanding and Approach to Illness and Health.* Jeffersonton, VA: Perelandra Center for Nature Research, 1988.

Index

Titchener, E.B., 22
trauma, effects of unhealed,
 294–97
traumatic events, 207–12
traumatic residue, symptoms of,
 296
trying too hard vs. just being, 285

U
unconscious empathy, mimicry
 and, 81–83

V
vicarious trauma, 13–14
 caregivers at risk of, 12, 173
 effects of, 80–81
 energetic boundaries and, 30
 example of, 85–86, 142
 media and, 146
 treating with Bach remedies,
  173
vision board, 249–52
visualization, 240–70, 289–90
 barriers to effectiveness of,
  264–69

benefits of, 265–66
example use of, 253–56
how it works, 243, 266
techniques, 256–64
to correct psychoenergetic
 reversal, 117
to counteract energy vampires,
 137
to improve memory, 243–46
types of, 242

W
Weil, Andrew, 266–67
Western medicine
 evolution of, 58–62
 limits of, 40–42
 talk therapy, 207, 215, 293, 297
Wolpe, Joseph, 219–20

Y
yoga, 122, 187, 202

ABOUT THE AUTHOR

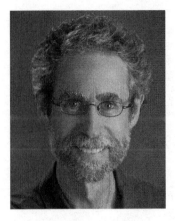 **Howard Brockman, LCSW, DCEP** is a psychotherapist and licensed clinical social worker who has been in private practice for over 31 years. He is the award-winning author of *Dynamic Energetic Healing®: Integrating Core Shamanic Practices With Energy Psychology Applications and Processwork Principles.* Through his training institute, Dynamic Energetic Healing® International™, he teaches other therapists and counselors how to reliably identify persistent unresolved emotional trauma responsible for current problem states and relationship issues. He provides an array of innovative therapeutic strategies for enabling rapid return to emotional balance. Self-care strategies with an emphasis on how to maintain interpersonal boundaries are a major emphasis of his work with clients and caregivers.

For more information about Howard's work, please visit his website at www.DynamicEnergeticHealing.com.

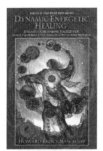

Dynamic Energetic Healing®

Integrating Core Shamanic Practices with Energy Psychology Applications and Processwork Principles

Author: Howard Brockman, LCSW

Synopsis: Howard Brockman introduces a new psychotherapy model that creatively integrates ancient spiritual healing practices with modern psychotherapy. Dynamic Energetic Healing® is an energy based psychotherapy model. The model assists readers to release and eliminate trauma caused by unidentified sources of anxiety, depression and relationship difficulties. Brockman's book explains the Dynamic Energetic Healing® model and its practical applications, along with seventeen in-depth case studies that illustrate the model's successful implementation.

Availability: Online through www.DynamicEnergeticHealing.com (paperback and PDF eBook), www.Amazon.com (paperback and Kindle), Apple's iBookstore (iPad and iPod) and www.BN.com (Barnes & Noble's Nook eReader).

Publishing Awards:

 October, 2006 Finalist in the "New Age: Non-Fiction" category of the "BEST BOOKS 2006" **National Book Awards** of www.USABookNews.com.

 May, 2007 **2007 Independent Publisher Book Award.** Silver IPPY award for 2007 National Categories in Psychology/Mental Health.

 May, 2007 **Eric Hoffer Award** for Excellence in Independent Publishing. www.HofferAward.com

 May, 2007 Finalist, 2007 **Nautilus Book Awards** in the Health & Healing category. www.Marilynmcguire.com

Endorsements:

"In his Dynamic Energetic Healing theory and methods, Howard Brockman creatively bridges shamanism and body oriented psychological healing practices to create new methods to heal trauma and help integrate body, mind, and spirit. This book is easily read and very practical for both therapists and clients."
– Arnold Mindell, PhD, author of *The Quantum Mind and Healing: How to Listen and Respond to Your Body's Symptoms.*

"The world of psychotherapy is in constant flux. Howard Brockman has brought a novel perspective to this field. His theoretical description demonstrates a deep knowledge of several healing traditions from various parts of the globe."
– Stanley Krippner, PhD, co-author of *Extraordinary Dreams and How to Work with Them*

"Dynamic Energetic Healing® helps to bridge the gap between Eastern and Western medicine, offering us new ways to approach client work and our common goal of planetary healing."
– Alberto Villoldo, PhD, author of *Shaman, Healer, Sage*

"Howard Brockman provides a wealth of information, creatively synthesizing ancient spiritual healing practices with modern psychotherapy to create a holistic approach to healing. This book contains powerful healing!"
– Sandra Ingerman, MA, author of *Soul Retrieval and Medicine for the Earth*

Library of Congress number: 2005903096
Hardcover ISBN 10: 0-9766469-3-5
Hardcover ISBN 13: 978-0-9766469-3-8
Paperback ISBN-10: 0-9766469-7-8
Paperback ISBN-13: 978-0-0766469-7-6

Contact Information:
Howard Brockman, LCSW
Columbia Press, LLC
1620 Commercial Street SE
Salem, Oregon 97302
voice: 503.370.4546
email: orders@DynamicEnergeticHealing.com
online: www.DynamicEnergeticHealing.com

Made in the USA
Lexington, KY
31 August 2016